Welcome to the ***"Gut Health Cookbook for Men: 115+ Recipes to Support Digestive Harmony and Energy"!*** This cookbook is your comprehensive guide to enhancing your digestive health through delicious and nourishing recipes tailored specifically for men.

Why This Cookbook?

Maintaining optimal gut health is crucial for overall well-being, energy levels, and even mental clarity. This cookbook is designed to help you achieve digestive harmony by providing over 115 recipes that focus on ingredients known for their gut-friendly properties. Whether you're looking to alleviate digestive discomfort, support a healthy microbiome, or simply improve your overall health, these recipes will empower you to make informed and nutritious food choices.

What You'll Find Inside

Inside this cookbook, you'll discover a variety of recipes carefully crafted to promote digestive wellness while satisfying your taste buds. From hearty breakfasts and satisfying lunches to wholesome dinners and nutritious snacks, each recipe is packed with ingredients chosen for their digestive benefits. You'll also find tips on ingredient selection, cooking techniques, and meal planning to help you integrate these recipes into your daily routine seamlessly.

Key Features:

- ***Digestive-Friendly Recipes:*** Explore over 115 recipes that incorporate gut-supportive ingredients such as fiber-rich foods, probiotics, and anti-inflammatory spices.

- ***Easy-to-Follow Instructions:*** Each recipe includes clear instructions, cooking tips, and nutritional information to guide you through preparing delicious meals that support digestive health.

- ***Variety of Dishes:*** Enjoy a wide range of recipes including soups, salads, main courses, desserts, and more, ensuring there's something for every meal and occasion.

- ***Nutritional Benefits:*** Learn about the nutritional benefits of key ingredients and how they contribute to digestive health and overall well-being.

- ***Lifestyle Tips:*** Discover practical lifestyle tips and habits that complement your dietary choices, enhancing your journey towards better digestive health.

Sample Recipes:

- Quinoa and Roasted Vegetable Buddha Bowl
- Salmon with Lemon and Dill Yogurt Sauce
- Turmeric Ginger Carrot Soup
- Greek Yogurt Parfait with Berries and Almonds
- Grilled Chicken Caesar Salad with Homemade Dressing

Start Your Journey

Whether you're looking to manage digestive issues, enhance your energy levels, or simply adopt a healthier lifestyle, "Gut Health Cookbook for Men: 115+ Recipes to Support Digestive Harmony and Energy" is your companion on this journey. By prioritizing your gut health with nutritious and delicious meals, you'll not only feel better physically but also cultivate habits that support long-term well-being. Here's to a healthier digestive system and a more vibrant you!

1. Greek Yogurt with Honey and Berries

Ingredient:

- 1 cup plain Greek yogurt
- 2 tbsp honey
- 1/2 cup mixed berries (such as blueberries, raspberries, blackberries)

Instructions:

1. Scoop the Greek yogurt into a bowl.

2. Drizzle the honey over the top of the yogurt.

3. Gently fold the honey into the yogurt until it is swirled throughout.

4. Top the yogurt with the mixed berries.

5. Serve immediately and enjoy!

This makes a delicious and healthy breakfast or snack. The creamy Greek yogurt paired with the sweetness of the honey and the freshness of the berries is a wonderful flavor combination. Feel free to adjust the amounts of honey or berries to your taste preferences.

2. Overnight Oats with Chia Seeds and Almond Milk

Ingredient:

• 1 cup rolled oats
• 1 tablespoon chia seeds
• 1 cup unsweetened almond milk
• 1 tablespoon maple syrup (optional)
• 1/2 teaspoon vanilla extract
• Pinch of cinnamon

Instructions:

1. In a medium•sized bowl, combine the rolled oats and chia seeds.

2. Pour in the almond milk and stir to combine.

3. If desired, add the maple syrup and vanilla extract, and stir again.

4. Cover the bowl and refrigerate overnight, or for at least 4 hours.

5. When ready to serve, give the mixture a stir and top with a sprinkle of cinnamon.

Why this recipe supports gut health for men:

1. Rolled Oats: Oats are a great source of soluble fiber, which can help promote healthy digestion and support the growth of beneficial gut bacteria.

2. Chia Seeds: Chia seeds are rich in fiber, omega•3 fatty acids, and antioxidants, all of which can contribute to a healthy gut microbiome.

3. Almond Milk: Unsweetened almond milk is a dairy•free option that is low in sugar and easy to digest, making it a gut•friendly choice.

4. Cinnamon: This spice has been shown to have anti•inflammatory properties and may help improve gut health.

This simple and delicious overnight oats recipe can be a great addition to a man's diet, providing a nutritious and gut•supporting breakfast option.

3. Avocado Toast on Whole Grain Bread

Ingredient:

- 2 slices of whole grain bread
- 1 ripe avocado, mashed
- 1 tablespoon olive oil
- 1 tablespoon lemon juice
- 1/4 teaspoon sea salt
- 1/4 teaspoon ground black pepper
- 1 tablespoon chopped fresh cilantro (optional)

Instructions:

1. Toast the whole grain bread until lightly golden.

2. In a small bowl, mash the avocado with a fork. Add the olive oil, lemon juice, salt, and pepper, and mix well.

3. Spread the avocado mixture evenly over the toasted bread slices.

4. Sprinkle the chopped cilantro on top, if using.

Why this recipe supports gut health:

1. Whole Grain Bread: Whole grains are rich in fiber, which can help promote healthy digestion and support the growth of beneficial gut bacteria.

2. Avocado: Avocados are a great source of healthy fats, fiber, and antioxidants, all of which can contribute to a healthy gut microbiome.

3. Olive Oil: Olive oil is a healthy fat that has been shown to have anti·inflammatory properties, which can be beneficial for gut health.

4. Lemon Juice: Lemon juice is a natural source of vitamin C and can help support the immune system, which is closely linked to gut health.

5. Cilantro (optional): Cilantro is a herb that has been shown to have antimicrobial properties and may help support a healthy gut.

This simple and nutritious avocado toast recipe can be a great option for men looking to support their gut health through their diet.

4. Smoothie with Spinach, Banana, and Kefir

Ingredient:

- 1 cup unsweetened kefir
- 1 cup fresh spinach leaves
- 1 ripe banana, frozen
- 1 tablespoon ground flaxseed
- 1 teaspoon honey (optional)
- 1/2 cup ice cubes (optional)

Instructions:

1. Add the kefir, spinach, frozen banana, and ground flaxseed to a high•speed blender.

2. Blend the ingredients until smooth and creamy.

3. If desired, add a teaspoon of honey and blend again to sweeten the smoothie.

4. If a thicker consistency is preferred, add the ice cubes and blend until smooth.

Why this recipe supports gut health:

1. Kefir: Kefir is a fermented dairy product that is rich in probiotics, which can help support a healthy gut microbiome.

2. Spinach: Spinach is a leafy green vegetable that is high in fiber, which can promote healthy digestion and support the growth of beneficial gut bacteria.

3. Banana: Bananas are a prebiotic food, meaning they contain fiber that feeds the good bacteria in your gut.

4. Flaxseed: Ground flaxseed is a great source of soluble fiber, which can help improve gut health and regularity.

5. Honey (optional): Honey has been shown to have antimicrobial properties and may help support a healthy gut.

This smoothie is a nutrient•dense and gut•friendly option that can be a great addition to a man's diet. The combination of probiotics, fiber, and antioxidants can help support overall gut health.

5. Scrambled Eggs with Spinach and Tomatoes

Ingredient:

• 3 eggs
• 1 tablespoon olive oil
• 1 cup fresh spinach, chopped
• 1/2 cup cherry tomatoes, halved
• 1 tablespoon grated Parmesan cheese (optional)
• Salt and pepper to taste

Instructions:

1. In a small bowl, whisk the eggs together until well combined.

2. Heat the olive oil in a non•stick skillet over medium heat.

3. Add the chopped spinach to the skillet and sauté for 1•2 minutes, until slightly wilted.

4. Pour the whisked eggs into the skillet and let them sit for 30 seconds to a minute, then use a spatula to gently scramble the eggs, incorporating the spinach as you go.

5. Once the eggs are almost fully cooked, add the halved cherry tomatoes and continue to scramble until the eggs are cooked through but still soft. Remove the skillet from the heat and sprinkle the Parmesan cheese over the top, if using. Season with salt and pepper to taste.

Why this recipe supports gut health:

1. Eggs: Eggs are a great source of protein, which can help support the growth of beneficial gut bacteria.

2. Spinach: Spinach is a leafy green vegetable that is high in fiber, which can promote healthy digestion and support the growth of beneficial gut bacteria.

3. Tomatoes: Tomatoes are a source of antioxidants, such as lycopene, which can help support a healthy gut microbiome.

4. Olive Oil: Olive oil is a healthy fat that has been shown to have anti•inflammatory properties, which can be beneficial for gut health.

5. Parmesan Cheese (optional): Parmesan cheese contains probiotics, which can help support a healthy gut microbiome.

This scrambled egg dish is a nutritious and gut•friendly breakfast option that can be a great way to start the day for men looking to support their digestive health.

6. Chia Seed Pudding with Fresh Fruits

Ingredient:

• 1/4 cup chia seeds
• 1 cup unsweetened almond milk
• 1 tablespoon maple syrup (or honey)
• 1/2 teaspoon vanilla extract
• 1/2 cup mixed fresh berries (such as raspberries, blueberries, and strawberries)
• 1/2 banana, sliced

Instructions:

1. In a medium·sized bowl, whisk together the chia seeds, almond milk, maple syrup, and vanilla extract until well combined.

2. Cover the bowl and refrigerate for at least 4 hours, or overnight, stirring occasionally, until the mixture has thickened to a pudding·like consistency.

3. When ready to serve, divide the chia seed pudding into two bowls or jars.

4. Top each serving with the mixed fresh berries and sliced banana.

Why this recipe supports gut health:

1. Chia Seeds: Chia seeds are rich in fiber, omega·3 fatty acids, and antioxidants, all of which can contribute to a healthy gut microbiome.

2. Almond Milk: Unsweetened almond milk is a dairy·free option that is low in sugar and easy to digest, making it a gut·friendly choice.

3. Maple Syrup (or Honey): These natural sweeteners can provide a touch of sweetness without the negative impact of refined sugars on gut health.

4. Berries: Berries are a source of polyphenols, which are plant compounds that can help support a healthy gut by promoting the growth of beneficial bacteria.

5. Banana: Bananas are a prebiotic food, meaning they contain fiber that feeds the good bacteria in your gut.

This chia seed pudding is a nutrient·dense and gut·friendly breakfast or snack option that can be a great addition to a man's diet.

7. Oatmeal with Flaxseeds and Blueberries

Ingredient:

- 1 cup rolled oats
- 1 1/2 cups unsweetened almond milk (or milk of your choice)
- 1 tablespoon ground flaxseeds
- 1/2 cup fresh or frozen blueberries
- 1 tablespoon honey (optional)
- Pinch of cinnamon

Instructions:

1. In a medium saucepan, combine the rolled oats and almond milk.

2. Bring the mixture to a simmer over medium heat, stirring occasionally, until the oats are cooked and the mixture has thickened, about 5•7 minutes.

3. Remove the saucepan from the heat and stir in the ground flaxseeds.

4. Top the oatmeal with the fresh or frozen blueberries.

5. Drizzle with honey, if desired, and sprinkle with a pinch of cinnamon.

Why this recipe supports gut health:

1. Rolled Oats: Oats are a great source of soluble fiber, which can help promote healthy digestion and support the growth of beneficial gut bacteria.

2. Flaxseeds: Ground flaxseeds are rich in fiber, omega•3 fatty acids, and antioxidants, all of which can contribute to a healthy gut microbiome.

3. Blueberries: Blueberries are a source of polyphenols, which are plant compounds that can help support a healthy gut by promoting the growth of beneficial bacteria.

4. Almond Milk: Unsweetened almond milk is a dairy•free option that is low in sugar and easy to digest, making it a gut•friendly choice.

5. Cinnamon: This spice has been shown to have anti•inflammatory properties and may help improve gut health.

This oatmeal dish is a nutritious and gut•supporting breakfast option that can be a great addition to a man's diet.

8. Quinoa Porridge with Almond Butter and Banana

Ingredient:

• 1 cup cooked quinoa
• 1 cup unsweetened almond milk
• 1 tablespoon almond butter
• 1 ripe banana, sliced
• 1 tablespoon chia seeds
• 1 teaspoon honey (optional)
• Pinch of cinnamon

Instructions:

1. In a small saucepan, combine the cooked quinoa and almond milk. Heat over medium heat, stirring occasionally, until the mixture is warm and creamy, about 5 minutes.

2. Remove the saucepan from the heat and stir in the almond butter until it's fully incorporated.

3. Transfer the quinoa porridge to a bowl and top with the sliced banana, chia seeds, and a drizzle of honey (if using). Sprinkle a pinch of cinnamon over the top.

Why this recipe supports gut health:

1. Quinoa: Quinoa is a gluten•free grain that is high in fiber, which can help promote healthy digestion and support the growth of beneficial gut bacteria.

2. Almond Milk: Unsweetened almond milk is a dairy•free option that is low in sugar and easy to digest, making it a gut•friendly choice.

3. Almond Butter: Almond butter is a source of healthy fats and fiber, both of which can contribute to a healthy gut microbiome.

4. Banana: Bananas are a prebiotic food, meaning they contain fiber that feeds the good bacteria in your gut.

5. Chia Seeds: Chia seeds are rich in fiber, omega•3 fatty acids, and antioxidants, all of which can support a healthy gut.

6. Cinnamon: This spice has been shown to have anti•inflammatory properties and may help improve gut health.

This quinoa porridge is a nutrient•dense and gut•friendly breakfast option that can be a great addition to a man's diet.

9. Fermented Sourdough Pancakes

Ingredient:

- 1 cup active sourdough starter
- 1 cup whole wheat flour
- 1 cup unsweetened almond milk
- 1 egg
- 1 tablespoon honey
- 1 teaspoon baking soda
- 1/4 teaspoon salt

Instructions:

1. In a large bowl, combine the active sourdough starter, whole wheat flour, and almond milk. Stir until well mixed. Cover and let the batter ferment at room temperature for 8·12 hours, or overnight.

2. After the fermentation period, whisk in the egg, honey, baking soda, and salt until the batter is smooth.

3. Heat a lightly oiled non·stick skillet or griddle over medium heat. Scoop about 1/4 cup of the batter onto the hot surface, forming pancakes.

4. Cook the pancakes for 2·3 minutes per side, or until golden brown. Serve the fermented sourdough pancakes warm, with your choice of toppings, such as fresh fruit, maple syrup, or yogurt.

Why this recipe supports gut health:

1. Sourdough Starter: The fermentation process used to create the sourdough starter introduces beneficial probiotics that can help support a healthy gut microbiome.

2. Whole Wheat Flour: Whole grains, like those found in the whole wheat flour, are high in fiber and can help promote healthy digestion.

3. Almond Milk: Unsweetened almond milk is a dairy·free option that is low in sugar and easy to digest, making it a gut·friendly choice.

4. Honey: This natural sweetener can provide a touch of sweetness without the negative impact of refined sugars on gut health.

5. Fermentation Process: The fermentation process used to create the sourdough batter can help increase the bioavailability of nutrients and promote the growth of beneficial gut bacteria.

10. Breakfast Burrito with Black Beans and Avocado

Ingredient:

• 1 (15 oz) can black beans, rinsed and drained
• 1 avocado, diced
• 2 eggs, scrambled
• 2 tablespoons salsa
• 1 whole wheat tortilla
• 1 tablespoon olive oil
• Salt and pepper to taste

Instructions:

1. In a small saucepan, warm the black beans over medium heat, stirring occasionally, until heated through.

2. In a separate skillet, scramble the eggs with a bit of olive oil, salt, and pepper.

3. Lay the whole wheat tortilla on a flat surface. Spread the warmed black beans down the center of the tortilla.

4. Top the black beans with the scrambled eggs and diced avocado.

5. Drizzle the salsa over the top. Fold the sides of the tortilla over the filling, then roll it up tightly to create a burrito.

Why this recipe supports gut health:

1. Black Beans: Black beans are a great source of fiber, which can help promote healthy digestion and support the growth of beneficial gut bacteria.

2. Avocado: Avocados are rich in healthy fats, fiber, and antioxidants, all of which can contribute to a healthy gut microbiome.

3. Whole Wheat Tortilla: Whole grains, like those found in the whole wheat tortilla, are high in fiber and can help support a healthy gut.

4. Salsa: Salsa is a source of various vitamins, minerals, and antioxidants that can help support gut health.

5. Olive Oil: Olive oil is a healthy fat that has been shown to have anti•inflammatory properties, which can be beneficial for gut health.

11. Kale and Quinoa Salad with Lemon Dressing

Ingredient:

• 1 cup cooked quinoa
• 4 cups chopped kale, stems removed
• 1 cup cherry tomatoes, halved
• 1/2 cup canned chickpeas, rinsed and drained
• 2 tablespoons sliced almonds
• 2 tablespoons freshly squeezed lemon juice
• 1 tablespoon extra•virgin olive oil
• 1 teaspoon Dijon mustard
• 1 teaspoon honey
• Salt and pepper to taste

Instructions:

1. In a large salad bowl, combine the cooked quinoa, chopped kale, halved cherry tomatoes, and rinsed chickpeas.

2. In a small bowl, whisk together the lemon juice, olive oil, Dijon mustard, and honey until well combined.

3. Drizzle the lemon dressing over the salad and toss gently to coat. Sprinkle the sliced almonds over the top of the salad.

4. Season the salad with salt and pepper to taste. Serve the kale and quinoa salad immediately, or refrigerate until ready to serve.

Why this recipe supports gut health:

1. Kale: Kale is a leafy green vegetable that is high in fiber, which can help promote healthy digestion and support the growth of beneficial gut bacteria.

2. Quinoa: Quinoa is a gluten•free grain that is high in fiber and protein, both of which can contribute to a healthy gut microbiome.

3. Chickpeas: Chickpeas are a good source of fiber and protein, which can help support a healthy gut.

4. Almonds: Almonds are a source of fiber, healthy fats, and antioxidants, all of which can contribute to a healthy gut.

5. Lemon Juice: Lemon juice is a natural source of vitamin C and can help support the immune system, which is closely linked to gut health.

12. Spinach and Strawberry Salad with Walnuts

Ingredient:

- 5 oz baby spinach leaves
- 1 cup fresh strawberries, sliced
- 1/4 cup raw walnuts, chopped
- 2 tablespoons balsamic vinegar
- 1 tablespoon extra•virgin olive oil
- 1 teaspoon Dijon mustard
- 1 teaspoon honey
- Salt and pepper to taste

Instructions:

1. In a large salad bowl, combine the baby spinach leaves, sliced strawberries, and chopped walnuts.

2. In a small bowl, whisk together the balsamic vinegar, olive oil, Dijon mustard, and honey until well combined.

3. Drizzle the dressing over the salad and toss gently to coat. Season the salad with salt and pepper to taste. Serve the spinach and strawberry salad immediately.

Why this recipe supports gut health:

1. Spinach: Spinach is a leafy green vegetable that is high in fiber, which can help promote healthy digestion and support the growth of beneficial gut bacteria.

2. Strawberries: Strawberries are a source of polyphenols, which are plant compounds that can help support a healthy gut by promoting the growth of beneficial bacteria.

3. Walnuts: Walnuts are a good source of fiber, omega•3 fatty acids, and antioxidants, all of which can contribute to a healthy gut microbiome.

4. Balsamic Vinegar: Balsamic vinegar has been shown to have antimicrobial properties and may help support a healthy gut microbiome.

5. Olive Oil: Olive oil is a healthy fat that has been shown to have anti•inflammatory properties, which can be beneficial for gut health.

This spinach and strawberry salad with walnuts is a delicious and gut•friendly option that can be a great addition to a man's diet.

13. Greek Salad with Fermented Feta

Ingredient:

• 1 head romaine lettuce, chopped
• 1 cucumber, diced
• 1 pint cherry tomatoes, halved
• 1/2 red onion, thinly sliced
• 1 cup kalamata olives, pitted and halved
• 1 cup fermented feta cheese, crumbled
• 2 tablespoons olive oil
• 1 tablespoon red wine vinegar
• 1 teaspoon dried oregano
• Salt and pepper to taste

Instructions:

1. In a large salad bowl, combine the chopped romaine lettuce, diced cucumber, halved cherry tomatoes, sliced red onion, and halved kalamata olives.

2. Sprinkle the crumbled fermented feta cheese over the top of the salad. In a small bowl, whisk together the olive oil, red wine vinegar, and dried oregano. Drizzle the dressing over the salad and toss gently to coat.

3. Season the salad with salt and pepper to taste. Serve the Greek salad immediately, or refrigerate until ready to serve.

Why this recipe supports gut health:

1. Fermented Feta Cheese: Fermented feta cheese contains probiotics, which can help replenish the good bacteria in your gut.

2. Olive Oil: Olive oil is a healthy fat that has been shown to have anti•inflammatory properties, which can be beneficial for gut health.

3. Red Wine Vinegar: Red wine vinegar has been shown to have antimicrobial properties and may help support a healthy gut microbiome.

4. Vegetables: The vegetables in this salad, such as romaine lettuce, cucumbers, and tomatoes, are high in fiber, which can help promote healthy digestion and support the growth of beneficial gut bacteria.

5. Olives: Olives are a source of polyphenols, which are plant compounds that can help support a healthy gut by promoting the growth of beneficial bacteria.

14. Beetroot and Arugula Salad with Goat Cheese

Ingredient:
- 4 cups baby arugula
- 2 medium beets, roasted and sliced
- 1/4 cup crumbled goat cheese
- 2 tablespoons toasted walnuts
- 2 tablespoons balsamic vinegar
- 1 tablespoon extra•virgin olive oil
- 1 teaspoon Dijon mustard
- 1 teaspoon honey
- Salt and pepper to taste

Instructions:
1. In a large salad bowl, combine the baby arugula, roasted and sliced beets, crumbled goat cheese, and toasted walnuts.

2. In a small bowl, whisk together the balsamic vinegar, olive oil, Dijon mustard, and honey until well combined.

3. Drizzle the dressing over the salad and toss gently to coat. Season the salad with salt and pepper to taste. Serve the beetroot and arugula salad immediately.

Why this recipe supports gut health:
1. Arugula: Arugula is a leafy green vegetable that is high in fiber, which can help promote healthy digestion and support the growth of beneficial gut bacteria.

2. Beets: Beets are a source of betalains, which are plant compounds that have been shown to have anti•inflammatory properties and may help support a healthy gut microbiome.

3. Goat Cheese: Goat cheese contains probiotics, which can help replenish the good bacteria in your gut.

4. Walnuts: Walnuts are a good source of fiber, omega•3 fatty acids, and antioxidants, all of which can contribute to a healthy gut microbiome.

5. Balsamic Vinegar: Balsamic vinegar has been shown to have antimicrobial properties and may help support a healthy gut microbiome.

6. Olive Oil: Olive oil is a healthy fat that has been shown to have anti•inflammatory properties, which can be beneficial for gut health.

15. Cabbage Slaw with Apple Cider Vinegar

Ingredient:

- 4 cups shredded green cabbage
- 1 cup shredded red cabbage
- 1 carrot, grated
- 1/4 cup thinly sliced red onion
- 2 tablespoons apple cider vinegar
- 1 tablespoon extra•virgin olive oil
- 1 teaspoon Dijon mustard
- 1 teaspoon honey
- Salt and pepper to taste

Instructions:

1. In a large bowl, combine the shredded green cabbage, shredded red cabbage, grated carrot, and thinly sliced red onion.

2. In a small bowl, whisk together the apple cider vinegar, olive oil, Dijon mustard, and honey until well combined.

3. Pour the dressing over the cabbage mixture and toss gently to coat. Season the slaw with salt and pepper to taste.

7. Cover and refrigerate the cabbage slaw for at least 30 minutes to allow the flavors to meld. Serve the cabbage slaw chilled or at room temperature.

Why this recipe supports gut health:

1. Cabbage: Cabbage is a cruciferous vegetable that is high in fiber, which can help promote healthy digestion and support the growth of beneficial gut bacteria.

2. Apple Cider Vinegar: Apple cider vinegar has been shown to have antimicrobial properties and may help support a healthy gut microbiome.

3. Olive Oil: Olive oil is a healthy fat that has been shown to have anti•inflammatory properties, which can be beneficial for gut health.

4. Dijon Mustard: Dijon mustard contains compounds that may have antimicrobial effects, which can help support a healthy gut.

5. Honey: This natural sweetener can provide a touch of sweetness without the negative impact of refined sugars on gut health

16. Broccoli and Cranberry Salad with Yogurt Dressing

Ingredient:

• 4 cups broccoli florets, chopped
• 1/2 cup dried cranberries
• 1/4 cup sliced almonds
• 1/4 cup plain Greek yogurt
• 2 tablespoons apple cider vinegar
• 1 tablespoon honey
• 1 tablespoon olive oil
• Salt and pepper to taste

Instructions:

1. In a large bowl, combine the chopped broccoli florets, dried cranberries, and sliced almonds.

2. In a small bowl, whisk together the Greek yogurt, apple cider vinegar, honey, and olive oil until well combined.

3. Pour the yogurt dressing over the broccoli mixture and toss gently to coat. Season the salad with salt and pepper to taste. Refrigerate the salad for at least 30 minutes to allow the flavors to meld. Serve chilled or at room temperature.

Why this recipe supports gut health:

1. Broccoli: Broccoli is a cruciferous vegetable that is high in fiber, which can help promote healthy digestion and support the growth of beneficial gut bacteria.

2. Cranberries: Cranberries are a source of polyphenols, which are plant compounds that can help support a healthy gut by promoting the growth of beneficial bacteria.

3. Greek Yogurt: Greek yogurt is a probiotic•rich food that can help replenish the good bacteria in your gut.

4. Apple Cider Vinegar: Apple cider vinegar has been shown to have antimicrobial properties and may help support a healthy gut microbiome.

5. Olive Oil: Olive oil is a healthy fat that has been shown to have anti•inflammatory properties, which can be beneficial for gut health.

This broccoli and cranberry salad with a creamy yogurt dressing is a delicious and gut•friendly side dish or snack that can be a great addition to a man's diet.

17. Lentil and Carrot Salad with Citrus Vinaigrette

Ingredient:

- 1 cup cooked lentils, cooled
- 2 carrots, grated
- 1/4 cup chopped fresh parsley
- Salt and pepper to taste
- 2 tablespoons olive oil
- 2 tablespoons freshly squeezed orange juice
- 1 tablespoon freshly squeezed lemon juice
- 1 teaspoon Dijon mustard
- 1 teaspoon honey

Instructions:

1. In a large bowl, combine the cooked and cooled lentils, grated carrots, and chopped parsley.

2. In a small bowl, whisk together the olive oil, orange juice, lemon juice, Dijon mustard, and honey until well combined.

3. Pour the citrus vinaigrette over the lentil and carrot salad and toss gently to coat. Season the salad with salt and pepper to taste.

4. Refrigerate the salad for at least 30 minutes to allow the flavors to meld. Serve the lentil and carrot salad chilled or at room temperature.

Why this recipe supports gut health:

1. Lentils: Lentils are a great source of fiber, which can help promote healthy digestion and support the growth of beneficial gut bacteria.

2. Carrots: Carrots are a source of prebiotic fiber, which can help feed the good bacteria in your gut.

3. Parsley: Parsley is a herb that has been shown to have antimicrobial properties and may help support a healthy gut microbiome.

4. Olive Oil: Olive oil is a healthy fat that has been shown to have anti•inflammatory properties, which can be beneficial for gut health.

5. Citrus Juices: The orange and lemon juices in the vinaigrette are a natural source of vitamin C, which can help support the immune system, which is closely linked to gut health.

6. Dijon Mustard: Dijon mustard contains compounds that may have antimicrobial effects, which can help support a healthy gut.

18. Mixed Greens with Fermented Vegetables

Ingredient:

• 5 oz mixed greens (such as spinach, arugula, and kale)
• 1/2 cup fermented vegetables (such as sauerkraut, kimchi, or pickled carrots)
• 1/4 cup toasted pumpkin seeds
• 2 tablespoons olive oil
• 1 tablespoon apple cider vinegar
• 1 teaspoon Dijon mustard
• 1 teaspoon honey
• Salt and pepper to taste

Instructions:

1. In a large salad bowl, combine the mixed greens and fermented vegetables.

2. In a small bowl, whisk together the olive oil, apple cider vinegar, Dijon mustard, and honey until well combined.

3. Drizzle the dressing over the salad and toss gently to coat. Sprinkle the toasted pumpkin seeds over the top of the salad.

4. Season the salad with salt and pepper to taste. Serve the mixed greens salad immediately.

Why this recipe supports gut health:

1. Mixed Greens: The leafy greens in this salad, such as spinach, arugula, and kale, are high in fiber, which can help promote healthy digestion and support the growth of beneficial gut bacteria.

2. Fermented Vegetables: Fermented vegetables, like sauerkraut and kimchi, are rich in probiotics, which can help replenish the good bacteria in your gut.

3. Pumpkin Seeds: Pumpkin seeds are a source of fiber, zinc, and antioxidants, all of which can contribute to a healthy gut microbiome.

4. Apple Cider Vinegar: Apple cider vinegar has been shown to have antimicrobial properties and may help support a healthy gut microbiome.

5. Olive Oil: Olive oil is a healthy fat that has been shown to have anti•inflammatory properties, which can be beneficial for gut health.

6. Dijon Mustard: Dijon mustard contains compounds that may have antimicrobial effects, which can help support a healthy gut.

19. Chickpea and Cucumber Salad with Mint

Ingredient:

• 1 (15 oz) can chickpeas, rinsed and drained
• 1 cucumber, diced
• 1/4 cup chopped fresh mint
• 2 tablespoons olive oil
• 2 tablespoons lemon juice
• 1 tablespoon apple cider vinegar
• 1 teaspoon Dijon mustard
• 1 teaspoon honey
• Salt and pepper to taste

Instructions:

1. In a large bowl, combine the rinsed and drained chickpeas, diced cucumber, and chopped fresh mint.

2. In a small bowl, whisk together the olive oil, lemon juice, apple cider vinegar, Dijon mustard, and honey until well combined.

3. Pour the dressing over the chickpea and cucumber salad and toss gently to coat. Season the salad with salt and pepper to taste. Refrigerate the salad for at least 30 minutes to allow the flavors to meld. Serve the chickpea and cucumber salad chilled or at room temperature.

Why this recipe supports gut health:

1. Chickpeas: Chickpeas are a good source of fiber, which can help promote healthy digestion and support the growth of beneficial gut bacteria.

2. Cucumber: Cucumbers are a source of water and fiber, both of which can help support a healthy gut.

3. Mint: Mint is a herb that has been shown to have antimicrobial properties and may help support a healthy gut microbiome.

4. Olive Oil: Olive oil is a healthy fat that has been shown to have anti•inflammatory properties, which can be beneficial for gut health.

5. Lemon Juice: Lemon juice is a natural source of vitamin C and can help support the immune system, which is closely linked to gut health.

6. Apple Cider Vinegar: Apple cider vinegar has been shown to have antimicrobial properties and may help support a healthy gut microbiome.

20. Avocado and Mango Salad with Lime Dressing

Ingredient:

• 1 ripe avocado, diced
• 1 ripe mango, diced
• 1 cup baby spinach leaves
• 1/4 cup chopped fresh cilantro
• 2 tablespoons olive oil
• 2 tablespoons freshly squeezed lime juice
• 1 teaspoon honey
• Salt and pepper to taste

Instructions:

1. In a large salad bowl, combine the diced avocado, diced mango, baby spinach leaves, and chopped cilantro.

2. In a small bowl, whisk together the olive oil, lime juice, and honey until well combined.
3. Drizzle the lime dressing over the salad and toss gently to coat.

4. Season the salad with salt and pepper to taste. Serve the avocado and mango salad immediately.

Why this recipe supports gut health:

1. Avocado: Avocados are a great source of healthy fats, fiber, and antioxidants, all of which can contribute to a healthy gut microbiome.

2. Mango: Mangoes are a source of prebiotic fiber, which can help feed the good bacteria in your gut.

3. Spinach: Spinach is a leafy green vegetable that is high in fiber, which can help promote healthy digestion and support the growth of beneficial gut bacteria.

4. Cilantro: Cilantro is a herb that has been shown to have antimicrobial properties and may help support a healthy gut.

5. Olive Oil: Olive oil is a healthy fat that has been shown to have anti•inflammatory properties, which can be beneficial for gut health.

6. Lime Juice: Lime juice is a natural source of vitamin C and can help support the immune system, which is closely linked to gut health.

21. Chicken and Vegetable Bone Broth

Ingredient:

• 3 lbs chicken bones (such as backs, necks, and feet)
• 1 onion, roughly chopped
• 3 carrots, roughly chopped
• 3 celery stalks, roughly chopped
• 4 cloves garlic, peeled
• 1 tablespoon apple cider vinegar
• 1 bay leaf
• 1 teaspoon whole black peppercorns
• 8 cups filtered water
• Salt to taste

Instructions:

1. Place the chicken bones, onion, carrots, celery, garlic, apple cider vinegar, bay leaf, and peppercorns in a large stockpot or slow cooker.
2. Pour the filtered water over the ingredients, making sure the bones are fully submerged.
3. Bring the mixture to a boil over high heat, then reduce the heat to low and let the broth simmer for 8•12 hours, skimming any foam or fat that rises to the surface.
4. Strain the broth through a fine•mesh sieve, discarding the solids.
5. Season the broth with salt to taste.
6. Allow the broth to cool, then transfer it to airtight containers and refrigerate for up to 1 week or freeze for up to 6 months.

Why this recipe supports gut health:

1. Chicken Bones: Chicken bones are a rich source of collagen, gelatin, and other nutrients that can help heal and soothe the gut lining.

2. Vegetables: The onions, carrots, and celery in the broth provide fiber, vitamins, and minerals that can support a healthy gut microbiome.

3. Apple Cider Vinegar: Apple cider vinegar has been shown to have antimicrobial properties and may help support a healthy gut microbiome.

4. Gelatin: The gelatin extracted from the chicken bones can help improve gut integrity and reduce inflammation.

5. Slow Cooking: The long simmering time helps extract the maximum amount of nutrients from the bones and vegetables, making the broth more gut•friendly.

22. Lentil Soup with Turmeric and Ginger

Ingredient:
- 1 cup dried brown or green lentils, rinsed
- 4 cups low•sodium vegetable or chicken broth
- 1 tablespoon olive oil
- 1 onion, diced
- 3 cloves garlic, minced
- 1 tablespoon grated fresh ginger
- 1 teaspoon ground turmeric
- 1 teaspoon ground cumin
- 1/4 teaspoon cayenne pepper (optional)
- Salt and black pepper to taste
- Chopped fresh parsley or cilantro for garnish (optional)

Instructions:
1. In a large pot, combine the rinsed lentils and broth. Bring to a boil over high heat.

2. Reduce the heat to medium•low, cover, and simmer for 20•25 minutes, or until the lentils are tender.

3. In a separate skillet, heat the olive oil over medium heat. Add the diced onion and sauté for 5•7 minutes, until translucent.

4. Add the minced garlic, grated ginger, turmeric, cumin, and cayenne (if using) to the skillet. Cook for 1•2 minutes, stirring constantly, until fragrant.

5. Transfer the sautéed onion and spice mixture to the pot with the cooked lentils. Stir to combine.

6. Season the soup with salt and black pepper to taste. Serve the lentil soup hot, garnished with chopped fresh parsley or cilantro, if desired.

Why this recipe supports gut health:
1. Lentils: Lentils are a great source of fiber, which can help promote healthy digestion and support the growth of beneficial gut bacteria.

2. Turmeric: This spice contains curcumin, a compound with anti•inflammatory properties that can help support a healthy gut.

3. Ginger: Ginger has been shown to have antimicrobial and anti•inflammatory effects, which can be beneficial for gut health.

23. Miso Soup with Tofu and Seaweed

Ingredient:

• 4 cups dashi (Japanese fish or vegetable stock)
• 2•3 tablespoons white or yellow miso paste
• 1 block firm or extra•firm tofu, cut into 1•inch cubes
• 2 cups thinly sliced shiitake mushrooms
• 1 cup thinly sliced napa cabbage
• 2 green onions, thinly sliced
• 2 tablespoons dried wakame seaweed, rehydrated in water

Instructions:

1. In a medium saucepan, bring the dashi to a gentle simmer over medium heat.

2. In a small bowl, whisk together the miso paste with a ladle of the hot dashi until smooth. Pour the miso mixture back into the saucepan and stir to combine.

3. Add the tofu, shiitake mushrooms, napa cabbage, and rehydrated wakame seaweed to the simmering broth. Cook for 2•3 minutes, just until the vegetables are tender.

4. Remove from heat and ladle the soup into bowls. Garnish with the sliced green onions.

5. Serve hot. Enjoy!

The key flavors in this miso soup come from the dashi broth and the umami•rich miso paste. The tofu, mushrooms, cabbage, and seaweed add heartiness and nutrition. It's a simple yet comforting Japanese soup.

24. Tomato and Basil Soup with Olive Oil

Ingredient:

• 2 tablespoons olive oil
• 1 onion, diced
• 3 cloves garlic, minced
• 1 (28 oz) can crushed tomatoes
• 2 cups vegetable or chicken broth
• 1/4 cup fresh basil leaves, chopped
• 1 teaspoon dried oregano
• 1/4 teaspoon red pepper flakes (optional)
• Salt and black pepper to taste
• Drizzle of high•quality extra virgin olive oil for serving

Instructions:

1. In a large saucepan or Dutch oven, heat the 2 tablespoons of olive oil over medium heat. Add the diced onion and sauté for 5•7 minutes until softened.

2. Add the minced garlic and cook for 1 minute until fragrant.

3. Pour in the can of crushed tomatoes and the broth. Stir to combine.

4. Bring the soup to a simmer and let it cook for 10•15 minutes, stirring occasionally, until slightly thickened.

5. Remove from heat and stir in the chopped fresh basil, dried oregano, and red pepper flakes (if using). Season with salt and black pepper to taste.

6. Ladle the tomato basil soup into bowls. Drizzle each serving with a bit of high•quality extra virgin olive oil.

7. Serve hot, with crusty bread if desired. Enjoy!

The olive oil adds a lovely richness and fruity flavor to this simple yet delicious tomato soup. The fresh basil brightens up the whole dish.

25. Butternut Squash Soup with Coconut Milk

Ingredient:

- 1 medium butternut squash, peeled, seeded, and cubed (about 4 cups)
- 1 onion, diced
- 3 cloves garlic, minced
- 1 tablespoon olive oil
- 1 teaspoon ground cumin
- 1 teaspoon ground coriander
- 1/4 teaspoon cayenne pepper (optional)
- 1 (13.5 oz) can full•fat coconut milk
- 4 cups low•sodium vegetable or chicken broth
- Salt and pepper to taste
- Chopped fresh cilantro for garnish (optional)

Instructions:

1. In a large pot or Dutch oven, heat the olive oil over medium heat. Add the diced onion and sauté for 5•7 minutes, until translucent.

2. Add the minced garlic, ground cumin, ground coriander, and cayenne pepper (if using) to the pot. Cook for 1•2 minutes, stirring constantly, until fragrant.

3. Add the cubed butternut squash, coconut milk, and vegetable or chicken broth to the pot. Bring the mixture to a boil.

4. Reduce the heat to low, cover the pot, and simmer for 25•30 minutes, or until the squash is very soft. Using an immersion blender or a regular blender, puree the soup until smooth.

5. Season the soup with salt and pepper to taste. Serve the butternut squash soup hot, garnished with chopped fresh cilantro if desired.

Why this recipe supports gut health:

1. Butternut Squash: Butternut squash is a source of fiber, vitamins, and antioxidants, all of which can contribute to a healthy gut microbiome.

2. Coconut Milk: Coconut milk is a rich source of medium•chain triglycerides (MCTs), which have been shown to have antimicrobial and anti•inflammatory properties that can benefit gut health.

26. Broccoli and Cauliflower Soup with Garlic

Ingredient:

• 2 tablespoons olive oil
• 1 onion, diced
• 4 cloves garlic, minced
• 1 head broccoli, florets chopped (about 4 cups)
• 1 head cauliflower, florets chopped (about 4 cups)
• 4 cups vegetable or chicken broth
• 1 cup unsweetened almond milk
• 1 teaspoon dried thyme
• Salt and black pepper to taste
• Chopped parsley for garnish (optional)

Instructions:

1. In a large pot or Dutch oven, heat the olive oil over medium heat. Add the diced onion and sauté for 5•7 minutes until translucent.

2. Add the minced garlic and cook for 1 minute until fragrant.

3. Add the chopped broccoli and cauliflower florets to the pot. Pour in the broth and almond milk. Stir in the dried thyme.

4. Bring the soup to a simmer and cook for 15•20 minutes, until the vegetables are very tender.

5. Using an immersion blender, carefully blend the soup until smooth and creamy. Alternatively, you can transfer the soup in batches to a regular blender.

6. Season the soup with salt and black pepper to taste.

7. Ladle the broccoli cauliflower soup into bowls and garnish with chopped parsley if desired. Serve hot, with crusty bread if desired.

This soup is packed with gut•friendly nutrients from the broccoli, cauliflower, and garlic. The fiber, antioxidants, and anti•inflammatory properties of these vegetables can help support a healthy gut microbiome, which is important for overall men's health. The almond milk also provides a creamy texture without dairy.

27. Carrot and Ginger Soup with Lemon

Ingredient:

• 2 tablespoons olive oil
• 1 onion, diced
• 3 cloves garlic, minced
• 1 tablespoon grated fresh ginger
• 1 lb carrots, peeled and chopped
• 4 cups vegetable or chicken broth
• 1 cup unsweetened almond milk
• 2 tablespoons freshly squeezed lemon juice
• Salt and black pepper to taste
• Chopped parsley for garnish (optional)

Instructions:

1. In a large pot or Dutch oven, heat the olive oil over medium heat. Add the diced onion and sauté for 5•7 minutes until translucent.

2. Add the minced garlic and grated ginger. Cook for 1 minute until fragrant.

3. Add the chopped carrots to the pot. Pour in the vegetable or chicken broth and the almond milk. Stir to combine.

4. Bring the soup to a simmer and cook for 20•25 minutes, until the carrots are very tender.

5. Using an immersion blender, carefully blend the soup until smooth and creamy. Alternatively, you can transfer the soup in batches to a regular blender.

6. Stir in the freshly squeezed lemon juice. Season the soup with salt and black pepper to taste.

7. Ladle the carrot ginger soup into bowls and garnish with chopped parsley if desired.

8. Serve hot, with crusty bread if desired.

The combination of carrots, ginger, and lemon in this soup provides a bright, flavorful, and nutrient•dense meal. The ginger and lemon help aid digestion, while the carrots are rich in fiber, vitamins, and antioxidants • all of which can support gut health.

28. Mushroom and Barley Soup

Ingredient:

- 1 tablespoon olive oil
- 1 onion, diced
- 3 cloves garlic, minced
- 8 oz mixed mushrooms (such as cremini, shiitake, and oyster), sliced
- 1 cup pearl barley, rinsed
- 6 cups low•sodium vegetable or chicken broth
- 2 cups water
- 2 bay leaves
- 1 teaspoon dried thyme
- Salt and pepper to taste
- Chopped fresh parsley for garnish (optional)

Instructions:

1. In a large pot or Dutch oven, heat the olive oil over medium heat. Add the diced onion and sauté for 5•7 minutes, until translucent.

2. Add the minced garlic and sliced mushrooms to the pot. Cook for an additional 3•5 minutes, stirring occasionally, until the mushrooms have softened.

3. Stir in the rinsed pearl barley, vegetable or chicken broth, water, bay leaves, and dried thyme. Bring the mixture to a boil.

4. Reduce the heat to low, cover the pot, and simmer for 45•60 minutes, or until the barley is tender.

5. Remove the bay leaves and season the soup with salt and pepper to taste.

6. Serve the mushroom and barley soup hot, garnished with chopped fresh parsley if desired.

Why this recipe supports gut health:

1. Mushrooms: Mushrooms are a source of prebiotic fiber, which can help feed the good bacteria in your gut.

2. Barley: Barley is a whole grain that is high in fiber, which can help promote healthy digestion and support the growth of beneficial gut bacteria.

3. Onions and Garlic: These aromatic vegetables contain prebiotic fibers that can help feed the good bacteria in your gut

29. Sweet Potato and Black Bean Soup

Ingredient:

• 2 tablespoons olive oil
• 1 onion, diced
• 3 cloves garlic, minced
• 2 medium sweet potatoes, peeled and cubed
• 1 (15 oz) can black beans, rinsed and drained
• 4 cups vegetable or chicken broth
• 1 teaspoon ground cumin
• 1 teaspoon chili powder
• 1/4 teaspoon cayenne pepper (optional)
• Salt and black pepper to taste
• Chopped cilantro for garnish (optional)

Instructions:

1. In a large pot or Dutch oven, heat the olive oil over medium heat. Add the diced onion and sauté for 5•7 minutes until translucent.

2. Add the minced garlic and cook for 1 minute until fragrant.

3. Add the cubed sweet potatoes, black beans, vegetable or chicken broth, cumin, chili powder, and cayenne (if using) to the pot. Stir to combine.

4. Bring the soup to a simmer and cook for 20•25 minutes, until the sweet potatoes are very tender.

5. Using an immersion blender, carefully blend the soup until it reaches your desired consistency. Alternatively, you can transfer the soup in batches to a regular blender.

6. Season the soup with salt and black pepper to taste.

7. Ladle the sweet potato and black bean soup into bowls and garnish with chopped cilantro if desired. Serve hot, with crusty bread if desired.

This soup is packed with gut•friendly ingredients like sweet potatoes, black beans, and garlic. The sweet potatoes are rich in fiber, vitamins, and antioxidants, while the black beans provide protein and prebiotics that can nourish the gut microbiome. The garlic also has antimicrobial properties that can support digestive health. This warming, comforting soup is a great option for men looking to support their gut health.

30. Kale and White Bean Soup

Ingredient:

• 2 tablespoons olive oil
• 1 onion, diced
• 3 cloves garlic, minced
• 1 bunch kale, stems removed and leaves chopped
• 1 (15 oz) can white beans, rinsed and drained
• 4 cups vegetable or chicken broth
• 1 teaspoon dried thyme
• Salt and black pepper to taste
• Grated Parmesan cheese for serving (optional)

Instructions:

1. In a large pot or Dutch oven, heat the olive oil over medium heat. Add the diced onion and sauté for 5•7 minutes until translucent.

2. Add the minced garlic and cook for 1 minute until fragrant.

3. Add the chopped kale leaves to the pot. Sauté for 2•3 minutes until the kale starts to wilt.

4. Pour in the vegetable or chicken broth and add the rinsed and drained white beans. Stir in the dried thyme.

5. Bring the soup to a simmer and cook for 15•20 minutes, until the kale is tender.

6. Using an immersion blender, carefully blend a portion of the soup to thicken it slightly, leaving some texture. Alternatively, you can transfer a cup or two of the soup to a regular blender, blend, and then return it to the pot. Season the soup with salt and black pepper to taste.

7. Ladle the kale and white bean soup into bowls. Top with a sprinkle of grated Parmesan cheese if desired. Serve hot, with crusty bread if desired.

This soup is a powerhouse of gut•supporting ingredients. Kale is rich in fiber, vitamins, and antioxidants that can nourish the gut microbiome. White beans provide protein and prebiotics that feed the beneficial bacteria in the gut. The garlic also has antimicrobial properties that can support digestive health. This hearty, nutrient•dense soup is a great option for men looking to improve their gut health.

31. Grilled Salmon with Asparagus

Ingredient:

• 4 (6 oz) salmon fillets
• 1 lb asparagus, trimmed
• 2 tablespoons olive oil, divided
• 1 teaspoon lemon zest
• 2 tablespoons freshly squeezed lemon juice
• 2 cloves garlic, minced
• 1 teaspoon dried dill
• Salt and black pepper to taste

Instructions:

1. Preheat grill or grill pan to medium•high heat.

2. In a shallow baking dish or resealable plastic bag, combine 1 tablespoon of the olive oil, lemon zest, lemon juice, garlic, and dried dill. Season with salt and pepper. Add the salmon fillets and turn to coat evenly. Let marinate for 15•20 minutes.

3. In a separate bowl, toss the asparagus spears with the remaining 1 tablespoon of olive oil. Season with salt and pepper.

4. Grill the salmon fillets for 4•6 minutes per side, or until cooked through and flaky. Transfer the salmon to a plate and cover to keep warm.

5. Grill the asparagus for 5•7 minutes, turning occasionally, until tender•crisp.

6. Serve the grilled salmon fillets immediately, topped with the grilled asparagus spears.

Optional Garnishes:
• Lemon wedges
• Chopped fresh parsley or dill

This simple yet flavorful dish features tender, flaky salmon paired with crisp, charred asparagus. The lemon, garlic, and dill marinade adds bright, herbal notes to the salmon. Grilling the salmon and asparagus together makes for an easy, healthy, and delicious meal.

32. Quinoa and Black Bean Stuffed Peppers

Ingredient:

• 4 bell peppers, halved lengthwise and seeded
• 1 cup cooked quinoa
• 1 (15 oz) can black beans, rinsed and drained
• 1 cup diced tomatoes
• 1/2 cup diced onion
• 2 cloves garlic, minced
• 1 teaspoon ground cumin
• 1 teaspoon chili powder
• 1/4 cup crumbled feta cheese (optional)
• Salt and pepper to taste
• Chopped fresh cilantro for garnish (optional)

Instructions:

1. Preheat your oven to 375°F (190°C).

2. Arrange the bell pepper halves in a baking dish or on a rimmed baking sheet.

3. In a medium bowl, combine the cooked quinoa, black beans, diced tomatoes, diced onion, minced garlic, ground cumin, and chili powder. Stir to mix well.

4. Spoon the quinoa and black bean mixture evenly into the bell pepper halves.

5. If using, sprinkle the crumbled feta cheese over the top of the stuffed peppers.

6. Bake the stuffed peppers for 25•30 minutes, or until the peppers are tender and the filling is hot.

7. Remove the stuffed peppers from the oven and season with salt and pepper to taste. Garnish with chopped fresh cilantro, if desired. Serve the quinoa and black bean stuffed peppers warm.

Why this recipe supports gut health:

1. Quinoa: Quinoa is a gluten•free grain that is high in fiber, which can help promote healthy digestion and support the growth of beneficial gut bacteria.

2. Black Beans: Black beans are a good source of fiber, which can help support a healthy gut microbiome.

3. Bell Peppers: Bell peppers are a source of vitamins, minerals, and antioxidants, all of which can contribute to a healthy gut.

33. Baked Cod with Lemon and Dill

Ingredient:

- 4 (6 oz) cod fillets
- 2 tablespoons olive oil
- 2 tablespoons freshly squeezed lemon juice
- 2 cloves garlic, minced
- 2 tablespoons chopped fresh dill, plus more for garnish
- 1/4 teaspoon paprika
- Salt and black pepper to taste
- Lemon wedges for serving

Instructions:

1. Preheat your oven to 400°F (200°C). Lightly grease a baking dish or line it with parchment paper.

2. In a small bowl, whisk together the olive oil, lemon juice, minced garlic, 2 tablespoons of chopped fresh dill, and paprika. Season with salt and black pepper.

3. Place the cod fillets in the prepared baking dish. Pour the lemon•dill mixture over the top, making sure to evenly coat the fish.

4. Bake the cod for 12•15 minutes, or until it flakes easily with a fork and is opaque throughout.

5. Remove the baked cod from the oven and garnish with additional chopped fresh dill.

6. Serve the cod immediately, with lemon wedges on the side.

This baked cod dish is a great option for supporting gut health in men. The cod is a lean, protein•rich fish that provides essential nutrients like omega•3 fatty acids, which can help reduce inflammation in the gut. The lemon and dill add bright, fresh flavors while also offering additional gut•friendly benefits.

Lemon is a good source of vitamin C, which can support the immune system and promote a healthy gut microbiome. Dill is rich in antioxidants and has been shown to have antimicrobial properties, which can help maintain a balanced gut flora.

Pair this baked cod with a side of roasted vegetables or a fresh salad for a complete, gut•healthy meal.

34. Chicken Stir•Fry with Mixed Vegetables

Ingredient:

- 1 red bell pepper, sliced
- 1 cup broccoli florets
- 1 cup sliced mushrooms
- 1 cup snow peas or snap peas
- 1 cup shredded cabbage
- 2 green onions, sliced
- 1/4 cup low•sodium chicken broth
- Salt and black pepper to taste
- Cooked brown rice, for serving
- 1 lb boneless, skinless chicken breasts, cut into 1•inch pieces
- 2 tablespoons low•sodium soy sauce
- 1 tablespoon rice vinegar
- 1 tablespoon sesame oil
- 2 tablespoons olive oil
- 3 cloves garlic, minced
- 1 tablespoon grated fresh ginger

Instructions:

1. In a medium bowl, combine the chicken, soy sauce, rice vinegar, and 1 tablespoon of the sesame oil. Toss to coat the chicken and let marinate for 15•20 minutes.

2. Heat the olive oil in a large wok or skillet over high heat. Add the marinated chicken and stir•fry for 3•4 minutes until lightly browned.

3. Add the minced garlic and grated ginger to the pan. Stir•fry for 1 minute until fragrant.

4. Add the sliced red bell pepper, broccoli florets, mushrooms, snow peas, and shredded cabbage. Stir•fry for 4•5 minutes, until the vegetables are tender•crisp.

5. Pour in the low•sodium chicken broth and the remaining 1 tablespoon of sesame oil. Toss everything together and cook for 2•3 minutes more, until the sauce has thickened slightly.

6. Remove from heat and stir in the sliced green onions. Season with salt and black pepper to taste. Serve the chicken stir•fry immediately over cooked brown rice.

This stir•fry is packed with gut•friendly ingredients like garlic, ginger, and a variety of vegetables. The chicken provides lean protein, while the vegetables offer fiber, vitamins, and antioxidants that can support a healthy gut microbiome. Serving it over whole grain brown rice adds more fiber to the meal. This dish is a great option for men looking to improve their digestive health.

35. Spaghetti Squash with Marinara Sauce

Ingredient:

- 1 medium spaghetti squash (about 3 lbs)
- 2 tablespoons olive oil
- 1 onion, diced
- 3 cloves garlic, minced
- 1 (28 oz) can crushed tomatoes
- 2 tablespoons tomato paste
- 1 teaspoon dried oregano
- 1/2 teaspoon dried basil
- Salt and black pepper to taste
- Grated Parmesan cheese for serving (optional)
- Chopped fresh basil for garnish (optional)

Instructions:

1. Preheat your oven to 400°F (200°C).

2. Cut the spaghetti squash in half lengthwise and scoop out the seeds. Place the squash halves cut•side down on a baking sheet lined with parchment paper.

3. Bake the spaghetti squash for 40•50 minutes, or until it's tender and easily shreds with a fork.

4. While the squash is baking, prepare the marinara sauce. In a large skillet or saucepan, heat the olive oil over medium heat. Add the diced onion and sauté for 5•7 minutes until translucent.

5. Add the minced garlic and cook for 1 minute until fragrant.

6. Pour in the crushed tomatoes and tomato paste. Stir in the dried oregano and basil. Season with salt and black pepper to taste.

7. Bring the marinara sauce to a simmer and let it cook for 10•15 minutes, stirring occasionally, until thickened.

8. Once the spaghetti squash is cooked, use a fork to shred the flesh into long, spaghetti•like strands. Serve the spaghetti squash strands topped with the warm marinara sauce. Garnish with grated Parmesan cheese and chopped fresh basil, if desired.

This dish is a delicious and healthy alternative to traditional pasta. The spaghetti squash provides a low•carb, gluten•free base, while the homemade marinara sauce is packed with flavor and nutrients.

36. Lentil and Spinach Curry

Ingredient:

- 1 cup dried red lentils, rinsed
- 4 cups low•sodium vegetable or chicken broth
- 1 tablespoon olive oil
- 1 onion, diced
- 3 cloves garlic, minced
- 1 tablespoon grated fresh ginger
- 1 tablespoon garam masala
- 1 teaspoon ground cumin
- 1/2 teaspoon ground turmeric
- 1/4 teaspoon cayenne pepper (optional)
- 4 cups fresh spinach leaves
- 1 (13.5 oz) can full•fat coconut milk
- Salt and pepper to taste
- Chopped fresh cilantro for garnish (optional)

Instructions:

1. In a large pot, combine the rinsed lentils and vegetable or chicken broth. Bring the mixture to a boil over high heat.

2. Reduce the heat to low, cover the pot, and simmer for 15•20 minutes, or until the lentils are tender.

3. In a separate skillet, heat the olive oil over medium heat. Add the diced onion and sauté for 5•7 minutes, until translucent.

4. Add the minced garlic and grated ginger to the skillet. Cook for 1•2 minutes, stirring constantly, until fragrant.

5. Stir in the garam masala, ground cumin, ground turmeric, and cayenne pepper (if using). Cook for an additional minute.

6. Add the cooked lentils, fresh spinach leaves, and coconut milk to the skillet. Stir to combine and let the mixture simmer for 5•10 minutes, or until the spinach is wilted and the flavors have melded.

7. Season the curry with salt and pepper to taste. Serve the lentil and spinach curry hot, garnished with chopped fresh cilantro if desired.

37. Tofu and Vegetable Stir•Fry

Ingredient:

- 1 block (14 oz) extra•firm tofu, cubed
- 2 tablespoons sesame oil, divided
- 2 cloves garlic, minced
- 1 tablespoon grated fresh ginger
- 1 red bell pepper, sliced
- 1 cup broccoli florets
- 1 cup sliced mushrooms
- 1 cup snow peas or snap peas
- 2 green onions, sliced
- 2 tablespoons low•sodium soy sauce
- 1 tablespoon rice vinegar
- 1 teaspoon sesame seeds (optional)
- Salt and black pepper to taste
- Cooked brown rice, for serving

Instructions:

1. In a large skillet or wok, heat 1 tablespoon of the sesame oil over medium•high heat. Add the cubed tofu and sauté for 5•7 minutes, until lightly browned on all sides. Transfer the tofu to a plate and set aside.

2. In the same skillet, heat the remaining 1 tablespoon of sesame oil. Add the minced garlic and grated ginger. Sauté for 1 minute until fragrant.

3. Add the sliced red bell pepper, broccoli florets, mushrooms, and snow peas or snap peas to the skillet. Stir•fry for 4•5 minutes, until the vegetables are tender•crisp.

4. Return the sautéed tofu to the skillet. Pour in the low•sodium soy sauce and rice vinegar. Toss everything together and cook for 2•3 minutes more, until the sauce has thickened slightly.

5. Remove from heat and stir in the sliced green onions. Season with salt and black pepper to taste. Serve the tofu and vegetable stir•fry immediately over cooked brown rice. Sprinkle with sesame seeds, if desired.

This stir•fry is packed with gut•friendly ingredients like tofu, garlic, ginger, and a variety of vegetables. Tofu is a great source of plant•based protein, while the vegetables offer fiber, vitamins, and antioxidants that can support a healthy gut microbiome. Serving it over whole grain brown rice adds more fiber to the meal. This dish is a delicious and nutritious option for men looking to improve their digestive health.

38. Turkey Meatballs with Zucchini Noodles

Ingredient:

For the Meatballs:
- 1 lb ground turkey
- 1/2 cup breadcrumbs
- 1/4 cup grated Parmesan cheese
- 1 egg, beaten
- 2 cloves garlic, minced
- 1 teaspoon dried oregano
- 1/2 teaspoon salt
- 1/4 teaspoon black pepper

For the Zucchini Noodles:
- 3 medium zucchinis, spiralized or julienned
- 2 tablespoons olive oil
- 2 cloves garlic, minced
- Salt and black pepper to taste

For Serving:
- 1 cup marinara sauce, warmed
- Grated Parmesan cheese (optional)
- Chopped fresh basil (optional)

Instructions:

1. Preheat your oven to 400°F (200°C). Line a baking sheet with parchment paper.

2. In a large bowl, combine all the meatball ingredients (ground turkey, breadcrumbs, Parmesan, egg, garlic, oregano, salt, and pepper). Mix well until fully incorporated.

3. Roll the turkey mixture into 1•inch meatballs and place them on the prepared baking sheet.

4. Bake the meatballs for 18•20 minutes, or until cooked through and lightly browned.

5. While the meatballs are baking, prepare the zucchini noodles. Heat the olive oil in a large skillet over medium heat. Add the minced garlic and sauté for 1 minute until fragrant.

6. Add the spiralized or julienned zucchini noodles to the skillet. Sauté for 3•5 minutes, just until the noodles are tender but still have a bit of bite. Season with salt and black pepper to taste.

7. To serve, place the zucchini noodles in a bowl and top with the baked turkey meatballs. Drizzle the warm marinara sauce over the top.

8. Garnish with grated Parmesan cheese and chopped fresh basil, if desired.

This dish is a delicious and healthy alternative to traditional pasta and meatballs. The zucchini noodles provide a low•carb, nutrient•dense base, while the turkey meatballs are a lean protein source.

39. Baked Sweet Potato with Chickpeas and Spinach

Ingredient:

• 4 medium sweet potatoes, scrubbed clean
• 1 (15 oz) can chickpeas, rinsed and drained
• 2 cups fresh spinach, chopped
• 2 tablespoons olive oil
• 2 cloves garlic, minced
• 1 teaspoon ground cumin
• 1/4 teaspoon cayenne pepper (optional)
• Salt and black pepper to taste
• Chopped fresh parsley for garnish (optional)

Instructions:

1. Preheat your oven to 400°F (200°C).

2. Pierce the sweet potatoes several times with a fork. Place them directly on the oven rack and bake for 45•60 minutes, or until they are tender when pierced with a fork.

3. While the sweet potatoes are baking, prepare the chickpea and spinach topping.

4. In a medium skillet, heat the olive oil over medium heat. Add the minced garlic and sauté for 1 minute until fragrant.

5. Add the rinsed and drained chickpeas to the skillet. Sprinkle in the ground cumin and cayenne pepper (if using). Season with salt and black pepper.

6. Cook the chickpeas for 3•4 minutes, stirring occasionally, until they are lightly browned.

7. Add the chopped fresh spinach to the skillet and sauté for 2•3 minutes, until the spinach is wilted.

8. Remove the baked sweet potatoes from the oven and let them cool for a few minutes.

9. Slice each sweet potato in half lengthwise. Scoop out the flesh, leaving a thin layer attached to the skin. In a bowl, mash the sweet potato flesh. Stir in the chickpea and spinach mixture until well combined.

10. Spoon the sweet potato and chickpea mixture back into the potato skins.Serve the stuffed sweet potatoes warm, garnished with chopped fresh parsley if desired.

40. Cauliflower Rice with Grilled Shrimp

Ingredient:

For the Cauliflower Rice:
• 1 head of cauliflower, cut into florets
• 1 tablespoon olive oil
• 1 clove garlic, minced
• Salt and black pepper to taste

For the Grilled Shrimp:
• 1 lb large shrimp, peeled and deveined
• 1 tablespoon olive oil
• 1 teaspoon paprika
• 1/2 teaspoon garlic powder
• 1/4 teaspoon cayenne pepper (optional)
• Salt and black pepper to taste

For Serving:
• Chopped fresh parsley or cilantro
• Lemon wedges

Instructions:

1. Preheat your grill or grill pan to medium•high heat.

2. To make the cauliflower rice, place the cauliflower florets in a food processor and pulse until the cauliflower is broken down into small, rice•like pieces.

3. In a large skillet, heat the 1 tablespoon of olive oil over medium heat. Add the minced garlic and sauté for 1 minute until fragrant.

4. Add the riced cauliflower to the skillet. Season with salt and black pepper. Sauté for 5•7 minutes, stirring occasionally, until the cauliflower is tender and lightly browned.

5. In a medium bowl, toss the shrimp with the 1 tablespoon of olive oil, paprika, garlic powder, cayenne (if using), and a pinch of salt and black pepper.

6. Grill the seasoned shrimp for 2•3 minutes per side, or until they are opaque and cooked through.

7. Serve the grilled shrimp over the cauliflower rice. Garnish with chopped fresh parsley or cilantro and lemon wedges.

This dish is a great option for supporting gut health in men. Cauliflower is a cruciferous vegetable that is rich in fiber, which can help promote a healthy gut microbiome. The shrimp provides a lean source of protein, while the spices and herbs add flavor and additional gut•friendly benefits.

The combination of the cauliflower rice and grilled shrimp makes for a nutritious, low•carb meal that can help support overall digestive health.

41. Roasted Brussels Sprouts with Balsamic Glaze

Ingredient:

• 1 lb Brussels sprouts, trimmed and halved
• 2 tablespoons olive oil
• Salt and black pepper to taste
• 2 tablespoons balsamic vinegar
• 1 tablespoon honey
• 1 clove garlic, minced
• 1 tablespoon chopped fresh parsley (optional)

Instructions:

1. Preheat your oven to 400°F (200°C). Line a baking sheet with parchment paper.

2. In a large bowl, toss the trimmed and halved Brussels sprouts with the olive oil. Season with salt and black pepper.

3. Spread the Brussels sprouts in a single layer on the prepared baking sheet.

4. Roast the Brussels sprouts for 20•25 minutes, tossing halfway, until they are tender and lightly browned.

5. In a small saucepan, combine the balsamic vinegar, honey, and minced garlic. Bring the mixture to a simmer over medium heat, stirring occasionally, until it thickens slightly, about 3•5 minutes.

6. Remove the roasted Brussels sprouts from the oven and transfer them to a serving bowl.

7. Drizzle the balsamic glaze over the roasted Brussels sprouts and toss to coat evenly. Garnish the Brussels sprouts with chopped fresh parsley, if desired. Serve the roasted Brussels sprouts with balsamic glaze warm.

The combination of roasted Brussels sprouts and the sweet•tangy balsamic glaze creates a delicious and nutritious side dish. Brussels sprouts are a cruciferous vegetable that is rich in fiber, vitamins, and antioxidants, which can help support a healthy gut microbiome.

The balsamic vinegar in the glaze also provides beneficial acetic acid, which can help promote the growth of beneficial gut bacteria. This simple yet flavorful dish is a great way to incorporate more gut•friendly vegetables into your diet.

42. Fermented Kimchi

Ingredient:

- 3 cloves garlic, minced
- 1 tablespoon grated fresh ginger
- 2 tablespoons Korean red pepper flakes (gochugaru)
- 2 tablespoons fish sauce
- 1 tablespoon sea salt

- 1 medium head napa cabbage, cored and chopped
- 1 cup daikon radish, peeled and julienned
- 1/2 cup carrots, peeled and julienned
- 1/2 cup green onions, chopped

Instructions:

1. In a large bowl, combine the chopped napa cabbage, julienned daikon radish, julienned carrots, and chopped green onions.

2. In a small bowl, mix together the minced garlic, grated ginger, Korean red pepper flakes, fish sauce, and sea salt.

3. Add the seasoning mixture to the vegetable mixture and use your hands to massage and mix everything together thoroughly, ensuring the vegetables are well coated.

4. Pack the seasoned vegetables into a clean, wide•mouth jar or fermentation crock, pressing down firmly to remove any air pockets.

5. Cover the top of the vegetables with a weight, such as a small plate or a fermentation weight, to keep the vegetables submerged in the brine that will form.

6. Cover the jar with a lid, airlock lid, or cheesecloth and let the kimchi ferment at room temperature (around 65•75°F) for 3•7 days, depending on your desired level of sourness.

7. Check the kimchi daily, pressing down on the vegetables to keep them submerged. Taste the kimchi after 3 days and continue fermenting until it reaches your preferred flavor.

8. Once the kimchi is fermented to your liking, transfer the jar to the refrigerator. The kimchi will continue to develop flavor as it's stored.

Enjoy the fermented kimchi as a side dish, topping for rice or noodles, or as an ingredient in various recipes.

Kimchi is a probiotic•rich fermented food that can greatly benefit gut health. The fermentation process introduces beneficial bacteria that can help balance the gut microbiome, which is important for overall men's health. The spices and vegetables in kimchi also provide fiber, vitamins, and antioxidants that support digestive function.

43. Steamed Broccoli with Lemon

Ingredient:

• 1 lb broccoli florets
• 2 tablespoons water
• 1 tablespoon olive oil
• 2 tablespoons freshly squeezed lemon juice
• 1 clove garlic, minced
• 1/4 teaspoon salt
• 1/8 teaspoon black pepper
• Lemon zest for garnish (optional)

Instructions:

1. In a steamer basket set over a saucepan of simmering water, steam the broccoli florets for 5•7 minutes, or until tender but still crisp.

2. Drain the steamed broccoli and transfer it to a serving bowl.

3. In a small bowl, whisk together the water, olive oil, lemon juice, minced garlic, salt, and black pepper.

4. Pour the lemon•garlic dressing over the steamed broccoli and toss to coat the florets evenly.

5. Garnish the broccoli with a light dusting of lemon zest, if desired.

6. Serve the steamed broccoli with lemon warm or at room temperature.

This simple steamed broccoli dish is a great option for supporting gut health in men. Broccoli is a cruciferous vegetable that is rich in fiber, which can help promote a healthy gut microbiome. The fiber in broccoli acts as a prebiotic, feeding the beneficial bacteria in the gut.

The lemon juice in this recipe provides additional gut•friendly benefits. Lemon is a good source of vitamin C, which can help support the immune system and reduce inflammation in the digestive system.

The garlic in the dressing also has antimicrobial properties that can help maintain a balanced gut flora. This steamed broccoli with lemon makes for a nutritious and delicious side dish or a light, gut•healthy meal when paired with a lean protein source.

44. Garlic Roasted Asparagus

Ingredient:

• 1 lb asparagus, trimmed
• 2 tablespoons olive oil
• 3 cloves garlic, minced
• 1/2 teaspoon salt
• 1/4 teaspoon black pepper
• 1 tablespoon lemon juice (optional)
• Grated Parmesan cheese for serving (optional)

Instructions:

1. Preheat your oven to 400°F (200°C). Line a baking sheet with parchment paper.

2. In a large bowl, toss the trimmed asparagus spears with the olive oil, minced garlic, salt, and black pepper until the asparagus is evenly coated.

3. Spread the seasoned asparagus in a single layer on the prepared baking sheet.

4. Roast the asparagus for 12•15 minutes, or until it is tender and lightly browned, stirring halfway through.

5. Remove the roasted asparagus from the oven and transfer it to a serving dish.

6. Drizzle the roasted asparagus with the lemon juice, if using.

7. Sprinkle the roasted asparagus with grated Parmesan cheese, if desired.

8. Serve the garlic roasted asparagus warm.

This simple roasted asparagus dish is a great way to enjoy the natural flavors of the vegetable. The garlic adds a savory, aromatic element, while the lemon juice (if used) provides a bright, tangy note.

Asparagus is a nutrient•dense vegetable that is rich in fiber, vitamins, and antioxidants, all of which can support a healthy gut microbiome. The roasting process also helps to enhance the natural sweetness of the asparagus.

This side dish pairs well with grilled or baked proteins, such as chicken, fish, or tofu. It's a quick and easy way to incorporate more gut•friendly vegetables into your meals.

45. Mashed Cauliflower with Olive Oil

Ingredient:

• 1 large head of cauliflower, cut into florets
• 2 tablespoons olive oil
• 2 cloves garlic, minced
• 1/4 cup unsweetened almond milk (or regular milk)
• 2 tablespoons grated Parmesan cheese (optional)
• Salt and black pepper to taste
• Chopped fresh parsley for garnish (optional)

Instructions:

1. In a large pot, bring a few inches of water to a boil. Add the cauliflower florets, cover, and steam for 8•10 minutes, or until the cauliflower is very tender.

2. Drain the steamed cauliflower and transfer it to a food processor or high•powered blender.

3. Add the olive oil and minced garlic to the food processor. Blend the cauliflower, oil, and garlic until smooth and creamy, scraping down the sides as needed.

4. Gradually add the unsweetened almond milk (or regular milk) while blending, until you reach your desired consistency.

5. If using, stir in the grated Parmesan cheese.

6. Season the mashed cauliflower with salt and black pepper to taste.

7. Transfer the mashed cauliflower to a serving bowl and garnish with chopped fresh parsley, if desired. Serve the mashed cauliflower warm.

This mashed cauliflower dish is a great alternative to traditional mashed potatoes, and it can help support gut health in men. Cauliflower is a cruciferous vegetable that is rich in fiber, which can help promote a healthy gut microbiome.

The olive oil in this recipe provides healthy fats that can also benefit gut health. Olive oil contains monounsaturated fatty acids and antioxidants that can help reduce inflammation in the digestive system.

The optional Parmesan cheese adds a creamy, savory element, while the garlic provides antimicrobial properties that can help maintain a balanced gut flora

46. Roasted Carrots with Thyme

Ingredient:

• 1 lb carrots, peeled and cut into 1·inch pieces
• 2 tablespoons olive oil
• 1 teaspoon dried thyme
• 1/2 teaspoon garlic powder
• Salt and black pepper to taste
• Chopped fresh parsley for garnish (optional)

Instructions:

1. Preheat your oven to 400°F (200°C). Line a baking sheet with parchment paper.

2. In a large bowl, toss the peeled and cut carrots with the olive oil, dried thyme, garlic powder, and a generous pinch of salt and black pepper.

3. Spread the seasoned carrots in a single layer on the prepared baking sheet.

4. Roast the carrots for 25·30 minutes, flipping them halfway through, until they are tender and lightly caramelized.

5. Remove the roasted carrots from the oven and transfer them to a serving dish.

6. Garnish the carrots with chopped fresh parsley, if desired.

7. Serve the roasted carrots warm.

This simple roasted carrot dish is a great option for supporting gut health in men. Carrots are a rich source of fiber, which can help promote a healthy gut microbiome. The fiber in carrots acts as a prebiotic, feeding the beneficial bacteria in the gut.

Additionally, the thyme used in this recipe has antimicrobial properties that can help maintain a balanced gut flora. Thyme is also a good source of antioxidants, which can help reduce inflammation in the digestive system.

Pair these flavorful, roasted carrots with grilled or baked protein, such as chicken or fish, for a complete, gut·healthy meal. The carrots can also be enjoyed as a side dish or added to salads and other vegetable·based dishes.

47. Sauteed Spinach with Garlic

Ingredient:

• 1 lb fresh spinach, washed and stems removed
• 2 tablespoons olive oil
• 3 cloves garlic, minced
• 1/4 teaspoon red pepper flakes (optional)
• Salt and black pepper to taste

Instructions:

1. In a large skillet or wok, heat the olive oil over medium heat.

2. Add the minced garlic to the hot oil and sauté for 1•2 minutes, until fragrant and lightly golden.

3. Add the fresh spinach leaves to the skillet. Use tongs or a spatula to gently toss and coat the spinach with the garlic•infused oil.

4. Cook the spinach, stirring occasionally, for 2•3 minutes, until it is wilted and tender.

5. If using, sprinkle the red pepper flakes over the sautéed spinach.

6. Season the spinach with salt and black pepper to taste.

7. Serve the sautéed spinach with garlic warm.

This simple sautéed spinach dish is a great way to incorporate more gut•friendly greens into your diet. Spinach is a nutrient•dense leafy green that is rich in fiber, vitamins, and antioxidants, all of which can support a healthy gut microbiome.

The garlic in this recipe also provides additional benefits for gut health. Garlic has antimicrobial properties that can help maintain a balanced gut flora, and it may also have anti•inflammatory effects in the digestive system.

This quick and easy sautéed spinach makes a great side dish or can be added to other meals, such as pasta, rice, or as a topping for proteins. It's a versatile and nutritious way to enjoy the gut•supporting benefits of spinach and garlic.

48. Quinoa Pilaf with Herbs

Ingredient:

- 1 cup uncooked quinoa, rinsed
- 2 cups low•sodium vegetable or chicken broth
- 1 tablespoon olive oil
- 1 onion, diced
- 2 cloves garlic, minced
- 1 cup diced mushrooms
- 1/2 cup diced bell pepper
- 1/4 cup chopped fresh parsley
- 2 tablespoons chopped fresh basil
- 1 tablespoon chopped fresh thyme
- Salt and black pepper to taste
- Lemon wedges for serving (optional)

Instructions:

1. In a medium saucepan, combine the rinsed quinoa and broth. Bring the mixture to a boil, then reduce the heat to low, cover, and simmer for 15•20 minutes, or until the quinoa is tender and the liquid is absorbed.

2. In a large skillet, heat the olive oil over medium heat. Add the diced onion and sauté for 5•7 minutes, until translucent.

3. Add the minced garlic and continue cooking for 1 minute, until fragrant.

4. Stir in the diced mushrooms and bell pepper. Sauté for 3•5 minutes, until the vegetables are tender.

5. Fluff the cooked quinoa with a fork and add it to the skillet with the sautéed vegetables. Stir to combine.

6. Remove the skillet from heat and stir in the chopped fresh parsley, basil, and thyme. Season with salt and black pepper to taste.

7. Serve the quinoa pilaf warm, with lemon wedges on the side if desired.

This quinoa pilaf is a great option for supporting gut health in men. Quinoa is a gluten•free, high•fiber grain that can help nourish the gut microbiome. The variety of fresh herbs used in this dish also provide additional gut•friendly benefits.

Parsley is a good source of antioxidants, while basil and thyme have antimicrobial properties that can help maintain a balanced gut flora. The sautéed vegetables, such as mushrooms and bell peppers, add fiber, vitamins, and minerals that can further support digestive health.

49. Sweet Potato Fries with Paprika

Ingredient:

- 2 lbs sweet potatoes, peeled and cut into 1/2•inch thick fry shapes
- 2 tablespoons olive oil
- 1 teaspoon paprika
- 1/2 teaspoon garlic powder
- 1/2 teaspoon salt
- 1/4 teaspoon black pepper

Instructions:

1. Preheat your oven to 400°F (200°C). Line a large baking sheet with parchment paper.

2. In a large bowl, toss the peeled and cut sweet potato fries with the olive oil, paprika, garlic powder, salt, and black pepper until the fries are evenly coated.

3. Spread the seasoned sweet potato fries in a single layer on the prepared baking sheet, making sure they are not touching each other.

4. Bake the sweet potato fries for 20•25 minutes, flipping them halfway through, until they are tender and lightly browned.

5. Remove the baked sweet potato fries from the oven and transfer them to a serving dish.

6. Serve the sweet potato fries with paprika warm.

These sweet potato fries are a delicious and nutritious alternative to traditional French fries. Sweet potatoes are a great source of fiber, vitamins, and antioxidants, which can help support a healthy gut microbiome.

The paprika and garlic powder add a flavorful seasoning to the fries, while the baking method results in a crispy exterior and tender interior without the need for deep frying.

Sweet potato fries make a great side dish or snack, and they pair well with a variety of main courses, from burgers to grilled meats and fish. Enjoy these tasty, gut•friendly fries as part of a balanced, healthy meal.

50. Mixed Bean Salad

Ingredient:

• 1 (15 oz) can kidney beans, rinsed and drained
• 1 (15 oz) can garbanzo beans (chickpeas), rinsed and drained
• 1 (15 oz) can black beans, rinsed and drained
• 1 cup diced cucumber
• 1/2 cup diced red onion
• 1/2 cup diced bell pepper (any color)
• 1/4 cup chopped fresh parsley
• 2 tablespoons olive oil
• 2 tablespoons red wine vinegar
• 1 tablespoon lemon juice
• 1 teaspoon Dijon mustard
• 1 clove garlic, minced
• 1/2 teaspoon dried oregano
• Salt and black pepper to taste

Instructions:

1. In a large bowl, combine the rinsed and drained kidney beans, garbanzo beans, and black beans.

2. Add the diced cucumber, red onion, bell pepper, and chopped fresh parsley. Toss to mix.

3. In a small bowl, whisk together the olive oil, red wine vinegar, lemon juice, Dijon mustard, minced garlic, and dried oregano. Season with salt and black pepper to taste.

4. Pour the dressing over the bean and vegetable mixture and toss gently to coat everything evenly.

5. Cover the salad and refrigerate for at least 30 minutes, or up to 4 hours, to allow the flavors to meld. Serve the mixed bean salad chilled or at room temperature.

This colorful and flavorful bean salad is a great option for a healthy, gut•friendly side dish or light main course. The combination of different beans provides a variety of fiber, protein, and complex carbohydrates that can nourish the gut microbiome.

The fresh vegetables, herbs, and tangy dressing add additional nutrients and antioxidants that can support overall digestive health. This salad is easy to prepare and can be made in advance, making it a convenient and nutritious choice for meals or snacks.

51. Greek Yogurt with Flaxseeds

Ingredient:

- 1 cup plain Greek yogurt
- 1 tablespoon ground flaxseeds
- 1 teaspoon honey (optional)
- Fresh berries or sliced fruit (optional)

Instructions:

1. In a small bowl, combine the plain Greek yogurt and ground flaxseeds. Stir to mix well.

2. If desired, drizzle the yogurt mixture with 1 teaspoon of honey for a touch of sweetness.

3. Top the yogurt with fresh berries or sliced fruit, such as blueberries, strawberries, or kiwi.

That's it! This simple, gut•healthy snack or breakfast is ready to enjoy.

The key ingredients in this recipe that support gut health for men are:

Greek Yogurt:
- Provides probiotics, which are beneficial bacteria that can help maintain a healthy gut microbiome.
- Contains protein, which is important for overall digestive function.

Flaxseeds:
- Rich in fiber, which can help promote regular bowel movements and feed the beneficial gut bacteria.
- Contains omega•3 fatty acids, which have anti•inflammatory properties that can benefit the gut.

The optional honey adds a touch of natural sweetness, while the fresh fruit provides additional fiber, vitamins, and antioxidants that can further support gut health.

This Greek yogurt with flaxseeds is a quick, easy, and nutritious snack or breakfast that can help support a healthy gut for men. It's a great option to incorporate into a balanced, gut•friendly diet.

52. Apple Slices with Almond Butter

Ingredient:

• 2 medium apples, cored and sliced
• 1/4 cup creamy almond butter
• 1 tablespoon honey (optional)
• 1 tablespoon chopped toasted almonds (optional)

Instructions:

1. Wash and core the apples, then slice them into thin wedges or rounds.

2. In a small bowl, stir together the almond butter and honey (if using) until well combined.

3. Arrange the apple slices on a serving plate or platter.

4. Dollop or drizzle the almond butter mixture over the apple slices, making sure to cover them evenly.

5. Sprinkle the chopped toasted almonds over the top, if using.

6. Serve immediately.

This simple snack or light dessert is a great way to enjoy the natural sweetness of apples paired with the creamy, nutty flavor of almond butter. The almond butter provides healthy fats, protein, and fiber, which can help keep you feeling full and satisfied.

The optional honey adds a touch of sweetness, while the toasted almonds provide a nice crunch and additional texture.

This apple and almond butter combination is a nutritious and delicious snack that can be enjoyed anytime. It's a great option for a quick and easy healthy treat or a simple way to incorporate more fruits and nuts into your diet.

53. Carrot and Celery Sticks with Hummus

Ingredient:

• 2•3 medium carrots, peeled and cut into sticks
• 2•3 celery stalks, cut into sticks
• 1 cup homemade or store•bought hummus

Instructions:

1. Wash and prepare the carrots and celery by cutting them into long, thin sticks.

2. Arrange the carrot and celery sticks on a serving platter or plate.

3. Place the hummus in a small bowl in the center of the platter.

4. Serve the carrot and celery sticks with the hummus for dipping.

Why this snack is great for gut health:

• Carrots are a good source of fiber, which helps promote healthy digestion and bowel movements.

• Celery is rich in antioxidants and contains compounds that can help reduce inflammation in the gut.

• Hummus is made from chickpeas, which are high in fiber and protein. The tahini in hummus also provides healthy fats.

• The combination of the crunchy vegetables and the protein•rich hummus makes for a satisfying and gut•friendly snack.

This simple snack is easy to prepare and provides a nutritious boost of fiber, vitamins, and minerals that support overall gut health. The hummus also adds a creamy, flavorful element that complements the fresh vegetables.

54. Mixed Nuts and Seeds

Ingredient:

• 1/2 cup raw almonds
• 1/2 cup raw walnuts
• 1/4 cup raw pumpkin seeds
• 1/4 cup raw sunflower seeds
• 2 tbsp chia seeds
• 2 tbsp ground flaxseeds
• 1 tsp sea salt

Instructions:

1. In a large bowl, combine the almonds, walnuts, pumpkin seeds, sunflower seeds, chia seeds, and ground flaxseeds. Toss to mix well.

2. Sprinkle the sea salt over the nut and seed mixture and stir to coat evenly.

3. Transfer the mixed nuts and seeds to an airtight container. Store at room temperature for up to 2 weeks.

Why this mix supports gut health for men:

• Almonds and walnuts are high in fiber, which helps promote healthy digestion.

• Pumpkin and sunflower seeds are rich in zinc, which is important for prostate health.

• Chia and flaxseeds are excellent sources of omega•3 fatty acids, which have anti•inflammatory benefits.

• The combination of nuts, seeds, and fiber helps feed the beneficial bacteria in the gut microbiome.

This nutrient•dense snack mix can be enjoyed by the handful or sprinkled on top of yogurt, oatmeal, or salads. It's a great way for men to support their overall gut and prostate health.

55. Kefir Smoothie

Ingredient:

- 1 cup plain kefir
- 1 cup frozen mixed berries (such as blueberries, raspberries, blackberries)
- 1 banana, frozen
- 1 tbsp honey (optional)
- 1/2 tsp vanilla extract
- 1/4 cup milk of your choice (dairy, almond, oat, etc.)

Instructions:

1. Add the kefir, frozen berries, frozen banana, honey (if using), and vanilla extract to a blender.

2. Pour in the milk of your choice and blend on high speed until smooth and creamy.

3. Pour the kefir smoothie into a glass and enjoy immediately.

Why this smoothie is great for gut health:

- Kefir is a fermented dairy product that is rich in probiotics, which help support a healthy gut microbiome.

- Berries are high in fiber, antioxidants, and prebiotic compounds that feed the beneficial gut bacteria.

- Bananas are a good source of resistant starch, which acts as a prebiotic to promote gut health.

- Honey contains antimicrobial properties and can help balance gut bacteria.

- The combination of probiotics, prebiotics, and anti•inflammatory ingredients make this smoothie a gut•friendly powerhouse.

This kefir smoothie is a delicious and easy way to incorporate more gut•supporting nutrients into your diet. It's a great breakfast or snack option that can help improve digestion and overall gut health.

56. Edamame with Sea Salt

Ingredient:

• 1 lb frozen edamame in the pod
• 1•2 tsp coarse sea salt

Instructions:

1. Bring a large pot of salted water to a boil. Add the frozen edamame and cook for 5•7 minutes until tender.

2. Drain the edamame and transfer to a serving bowl.

3. Sprinkle the coarse sea salt over the hot edamame and toss to coat evenly.

4. Serve the edamame warm, providing small dishes for the guests to discard the empty pods.

The key is to use a good quality coarse sea salt to season the edamame. The warm, salty edamame pods make for a tasty and healthy snack or appetizer. Enjoy!

57. Fermented Pickles

Ingredient:
- 4•5 medium cucumbers, sliced into spears or chips
- 3 cloves garlic, peeled and halved
- 2 tsp dill seeds
- 1 tsp black peppercorns
- 1 tbsp sea salt
- 3 cups filtered water

Instructions:
1. In a clean, wide•mouth mason jar, layer the cucumber spears, garlic, dill seeds, and peppercorns.

2. Dissolve the sea salt in the filtered water to make a brine. Pour the brine over the cucumbers, making sure they are fully submerged.

3. Cover the jar with a tight•fitting lid or airlock lid. Allow to ferment at room temperature (65•75°F) for 3•5 days, checking daily and skimming off any scum that forms.

4. Once the pickles have reached your desired sourness, transfer the jar to the refrigerator. The pickles will continue to ferment slowly at a cooler temperature.

5. Enjoy the fermented pickles as a snack or side dish. They will keep for several months in the fridge.

Why fermented pickles support gut health for men:
- The fermentation process increases the probiotic content, which helps populate the gut with beneficial bacteria.

- Cucumbers are high in fiber, which feeds the gut microbiome and promotes regular bowel movements.

- Garlic contains antimicrobial compounds that can help balance gut flora and reduce inflammation.

- The combination of probiotics, fiber, and anti•inflammatory properties make fermented pickles a great gut•supporting food for men.

Incorporating fermented foods like these pickles into the diet can be especially beneficial for men's gut and overall health. The probiotics and other nutrients help maintain a healthy digestive system.

58. *Sliced Bell Peppers with Guacamole*

Ingredient:
• 2 ripe avocados, pitted and mashed
• 1/4 cup diced red onion
• 2 tbsp chopped cilantro
• 1 tbsp lime juice
• 1 tsp minced garlic
• 1/2 tsp sea salt
• 1/4 tsp ground cumin
• 2•3 bell peppers, sliced into strips (any color)

Instructions:
1. In a medium bowl, mash the avocados with a fork until slightly chunky.

2. Stir in the diced red onion, chopped cilantro, lime juice, minced garlic, sea salt, and ground cumin. Mix well to combine.

3. Arrange the sliced bell pepper strips on a serving platter.

4. Scoop the guacamole into a small bowl and place it in the center of the platter.

5. Serve the sliced bell peppers with the guacamole for dipping.

Why this snack supports gut health for men:
• Bell peppers are high in fiber, vitamins, and antioxidants that support overall gut health.

• Avocados are rich in healthy monounsaturated fats, fiber, and prebiotic compounds that nourish the gut microbiome.

• Onions, garlic, and cilantro contain compounds that have anti•inflammatory and antimicrobial effects, which can help maintain a balanced gut.

• The combination of the crunchy bell peppers and creamy guacamole provides a satisfying and nutrient•dense snack.

This simple yet flavorful snack is a great way for men to get a boost of gut•supporting nutrients. The fiber, healthy fats, and antioxidants make it a nutritious choice.

59. Baked Kale Chips

Ingredient:
• 1 bunch kale, washed and stems removed
• 1 tbsp olive oil
• 1 tsp sea salt

Instructions:
1. Preheat your oven to 325°F (165°C).

2. Tear the kale leaves into bite•sized pieces and pat them dry with a clean towel or paper towels.

3. Place the kale pieces in a large bowl and drizzle with the olive oil. Use your hands to massage the oil into the kale, making sure all the leaves are evenly coated.

4. Spread the kale pieces out in a single layer on a large baking sheet lined with parchment paper.

5. Sprinkle the sea salt evenly over the kale.

6. Bake for 12•15 minutes, flipping the kale halfway through, until the leaves are crispy and lightly browned. Remove the kale chips from the oven and let them cool completely before serving.

Why baked kale chips support gut health for men:
• Kale is high in fiber, which helps promote regular bowel movements and a healthy gut microbiome.

• Kale is also rich in antioxidants and anti•inflammatory compounds that can help reduce gut inflammation.

• The baking process concentrates the nutrients in the kale, making them more readily available for absorption.

• Kale chips make for a satisfying, crunchy snack that can help curb cravings for less healthy options.

Incorporating these nutrient•dense kale chips into your diet is an easy way for men to support their gut health. The fiber, antioxidants, and anti•inflammatory properties make kale a great choice for promoting overall digestive wellness.

60. Blueberry and Almond Parfait

Ingredient:

• 1 cup plain Greek yogurt
• 1/2 cup fresh or frozen blueberries
• 2 tablespoons sliced almonds
• 1 tablespoon honey (optional)

Instructions:

1. In a parfait glass or small bowl, layer half of the Greek yogurt.

2. Top the yogurt with half of the blueberries.

3. Sprinkle half of the sliced almonds over the blueberries.

4. Repeat the layers, ending with the remaining yogurt, blueberries, and almonds.

5. If desired, drizzle the parfait with 1 tablespoon of honey. Serve chilled or at room temperature.

This Blueberry and Almond Parfait is a delicious and gut•healthy treat that can be enjoyed as a snack or light dessert.

The key ingredients that support gut health for men are:

Greek Yogurt:
• Provides probiotics, which are beneficial bacteria that can help maintain a healthy gut microbiome.
• Contains protein, which is important for overall digestive function.

Blueberries:
• Rich in fiber, which can help promote regular bowel movements and feed the beneficial gut bacteria.
• Contains antioxidants that can help reduce inflammation in the digestive system.

The optional honey adds a touch of natural sweetness, which can make this parfait more appealing to some.

This Blueberry and Almond Parfait is a simple, yet nutrient•dense treat that can be easily incorporated into a gut•friendly diet for men. The combination of probiotics, fiber, and antioxidants makes it a great choice for supporting overall digestive health.

61. Sauerkraut with Carrots

Ingredient:

• 1 head green cabbage, shredded (about 4 cups)
• 2 carrots, grated (about 1 cup)
• 1 tbsp sea salt
• Filtered water

Instructions:

1. In a large bowl, combine the shredded cabbage and grated carrots. Sprinkle the sea salt over the top and use your hands to massage the salt into the vegetables, squeezing and kneading for 5•10 minutes until the vegetables start to release their juices.

2. Pack the salted cabbage and carrot mixture into a clean, wide•mouth mason jar, pressing down firmly to remove any air pockets. The vegetables should be fully submerged in their own juices.

3. If needed, add a bit of filtered water to the jar to ensure the vegetables are covered. Leave about 1•2 inches of headspace at the top.

4. Cover the jar with an airlock lid or a regular lid with a small gap to allow gases to escape during fermentation.

5. Let the sauerkraut ferment at room temperature (65•75°F) for 4•6 weeks, checking it periodically and skimming off any scum that forms on the surface.

6. Once the sauerkraut has reached your desired sourness, transfer the jar to the refrigerator. The fermentation will slow down at the cooler temperature.

7. Enjoy the sauerkraut with carrots as a side dish, topping, or condiment. It will keep for several months in the fridge.

The addition of carrots to this sauerkraut recipe provides extra fiber, vitamins, and natural sweetness to balance the sourness of the fermented cabbage. This gut•friendly probiotic food is a great way to support digestive health.

62. Kombucha

Ingredient:

- Black tea or green tea
- Sugar
- SCOBY (Symbiotic Culture of Bacteria and Yeast)
- Starter kombucha liquid

Instructions:

1. Brew a strong batch of black or green tea and let it cool to room temperature. Stir in sugar until dissolved.

2. Add the SCOBY and starter kombucha liquid to the sweetened tea. Cover the container with a breathable cloth or coffee filter.

3. Allow the kombucha to ferment at room temperature for 7•14 days, tasting it periodically. The longer it ferments, the less sweet and more vinegary it will become.

4. Once it reaches your desired flavor, remove the SCOBY and pour the kombucha into bottles for a second fermentation. You can add fruit juice or other flavorings at this stage.

5. Let the bottled kombucha sit at room temperature for 2•7 more days to build up carbonation. Then refrigerate.

Tips:

- Use a glass, ceramic or food•grade plastic container for fermenting.

- Make sure to keep the SCOBY healthy by feeding it regularly.

- Experiment with different tea blends, fruit juices and flavorings.

- Be patient • kombucha takes time to develop its signature tart, effervescent flavor.

63. Fermented Carrots

Ingredient:

- 1 lb carrots, peeled and cut into sticks or coins
- 2 cloves garlic, peeled and sliced
- 1 tbsp sea salt
- 1 cup filtered water
- 1 tbsp whey (optional)

Instructions:

1. In a clean, wide•mouth mason jar, layer the carrot sticks and garlic slices.

2. In a separate bowl, dissolve the salt in the filtered water to make a brine.

3. Pour the brine over the carrots, making sure they are fully submerged. If needed, weigh down the carrots with a small plate or weight to keep them under the brine.

4. If using whey, stir it into the brine. The whey will help kickstart the fermentation.

5. Cover the jar with a tight•fitting lid or airlock lid. Allow to ferment at room temperature (60•75°F) for 5•10 days, checking periodically. The carrots should become crisp and tangy when ready.

6. Once fermented to your liking, transfer the jar to the refrigerator. The carrots will keep for several months.

Tips:
- Use fresh, crunchy carrots for best texture.
- Add other spices like peppercorns, dill, or chili peppers for extra flavor.
- Taste the carrots after 5 days and continue fermenting to reach your desired sourness.
- Burp the jar daily to release built•up gases.

64. Fermented Beets

Ingredient:
• 3•4 medium beets, peeled and sliced or cubed
• 3 cloves garlic, peeled and sliced
• 1 tbsp sea salt
• 3 cups filtered water

Instructions:
1. In a clean, wide•mouth mason jar, layer the sliced or cubed beets and garlic cloves.

2. Dissolve the sea salt in the filtered water to create a brine. Pour the brine over the beets, making sure they are fully submerged.

3. Cover the jar with an airlock lid or a regular lid with a small gap to allow gases to escape during fermentation.

4. Let the beets ferment at room temperature (65•75°F) for 4•7 days, checking daily and skimming off any scum that forms.

5. Once the beets have reached your desired level of sourness, transfer the jar to the refrigerator. The fermentation will slow down at the cooler temperature.

6. Enjoy the fermented beets as a side dish, snack, or added to salads. They will keep for several months in the fridge.

Why fermented beets support gut health for men:
• Beets are a great source of fiber, which helps promote regular bowel movements and a healthy gut microbiome.

• The fermentation process increases the probiotic content of the beets, providing beneficial bacteria for the gut.

• Beets are rich in antioxidants and anti•inflammatory compounds that can help reduce inflammation in the digestive system.

• The combination of fiber, probiotics, and anti•inflammatory properties make fermented beets a powerful gut•supporting food for men.

Incorporating fermented beets into the diet can be an excellent way for men to support their overall gut health and digestion. The probiotics, fiber, and other nutrients in this fermented vegetable can help maintain a balanced gut microbiome.

65. Tempeh Stir•Fry

Ingredient:
• 8 oz tempeh, cut into 1•inch cubes
• 2 tbsp coconut oil
• 1 red bell pepper, sliced
• 1 cup sliced mushrooms
• 2 cups chopped kale
• 3 cloves garlic, minced
• 1 tbsp grated ginger
• 2 tbsp tamari or soy sauce
• 1 tbsp rice vinegar
• 1 tsp sesame oil
• Salt and pepper to taste
• Cooked brown rice, for serving

Instructions:
1. In a large skillet or wok, heat the coconut oil over medium•high heat.

2. Add the tempeh cubes and cook for 3•4 minutes per side, until lightly browned. Transfer to a plate.

3. In the same pan, add the bell pepper, mushrooms, and kale. Sauté for 3•4 minutes until the vegetables are tender.

4. Stir in the garlic and ginger and cook for 1 minute until fragrant.

5. Add the cooked tempeh back to the pan. Pour in the tamari, rice vinegar, and sesame oil. Toss everything together and cook for 2•3 minutes.

6. Season with salt and pepper to taste. Serve the tempeh stir•fry over a bed of cooked brown rice.

Why this tempeh stir•fry supports gut health for men:
• Tempeh is a fermented soy product that is rich in probiotics, which support a healthy gut microbiome.

• Kale is high in fiber, which helps promote regular bowel movements and digestive regularity.

• Bell peppers and mushrooms contain antioxidants and anti•inflammatory compounds that can help reduce gut inflammation.

66. Natto with Rice

Ingredient:

- 1 package natto (fermented soybeans)
- 1 cup cooked short•grain rice
- 1 tsp soy sauce
- 1 tsp mustard (optional)
- Chopped scallions or nori for garnish (optional)

Instructions:

1. In a bowl, gently mix together the natto, cooked rice, soy sauce, and mustard (if using) until well combined.

2. Serve the natto and rice mixture warm, garnished with chopped scallions or nori if desired.

Why is this a good gut health option for men?

Natto is a traditional Japanese food made from fermented soybeans. It's an excellent source of probiotics, which are beneficial bacteria that support a healthy gut microbiome. A healthy gut is important for overall health, including immune function, nutrient absorption, and even mental well•being.

For men specifically, natto may help:

- Improve testosterone levels • Natto contains nattokinase, an enzyme that can help increase testosterone production.

- Reduce inflammation • The probiotics in natto have anti•inflammatory effects, which can be beneficial for men's health.

- Support prostate health • The probiotics in natto may help prevent prostate issues.

- Boost energy and libido • The nutrients in natto, like vitamin K2, can help increase energy and sexual function.

Pairing the natto with rice provides a balanced meal with complex carbs to fuel the body. The soy sauce and optional mustard add flavor and additional health benefits

67. Fermented Jalapeños

Ingredient:
- 1 lb fresh jalapeño peppers, sliced into rings
- 3 cloves garlic, peeled and sliced
- 1 tbsp sea salt
- 3 cups filtered water

Instructions:

1. In a clean, wide•mouth mason jar, layer the sliced jalapeños and garlic.

2. Dissolve the sea salt in the filtered water to create a brine.

3. Pour the brine over the jalapeños, making sure they are fully submerged.

4. Cover the jar with an airlock lid or a regular lid with a small gap to allow gases to escape during fermentation.

5. Let the jalapeños ferment at room temperature (65•75°F) for 4•7 days, checking daily and skimming off any scum that forms.

6. Once the jalapeños have reached your desired level of sourness and spiciness, transfer the jar to the refrigerator. The fermentation will slow down at the cooler temperature.

7. Enjoy the fermented jalapeños as a condiment, topping, or snack. They will keep for several months in the fridge.

Why fermented jalapeños support gut health for men:
- Jalapeños are rich in capsaicin, which has anti•inflammatory properties that can help reduce gut inflammation.

- The fermentation process increases the probiotic content of the jalapeños, providing beneficial bacteria for the gut.

- Jalapeños also contain fiber, which helps promote regular bowel movements and a healthy gut microbiome. The combination of probiotics, anti•inflammatory compounds, and fiber make fermented jalapeños a great gut•supporting food for men.

Incorporating fermented jalapeños into the diet can be an excellent way for men to support their overall gut health and digestion. The probiotics, anti•inflammatory properties, and fiber in this fermented condiment can help maintain a balanced gut microbiome.

68. Yogurt Parfait with Granola

Ingredient:

• 1 cup plain Greek yogurt
• 1/2 cup homemade granola
• 1/2 cup fresh berries (such as blueberries, raspberries, or strawberries)
• 1 tbsp honey (optional)

Instructions:

1. In a parfait glass or bowl, layer half of the yogurt on the bottom.

2. Top the yogurt with half of the granola and half of the fresh berries.

3. Repeat the layers, ending with the remaining yogurt, granola, and berries.

4. Drizzle the honey over the top, if using.

Why is this a good gut health option for men?

1. Yogurt: Plain Greek yogurt is an excellent source of probiotics, which are beneficial bacteria that support a healthy gut microbiome. A healthy gut is important for overall health, including immune function, nutrient absorption, and even mental well•being.

2. Granola: Homemade granola provides fiber, which helps feed the good bacteria in the gut. Fiber is essential for maintaining a balanced gut flora.

3. Berries: Berries are rich in antioxidants and polyphenols, which can help reduce inflammation and support a healthy gut.

For men specifically, this yogurt parfait with granola can help:

• Improve testosterone levels: The probiotics in the yogurt may help increase testosterone production.

• Reduce inflammation: The antioxidants and fiber in the granola and berries have anti•inflammatory effects, which can be beneficial for men's health.

• Support prostate health: The probiotics and antioxidants in this dish may help prevent prostate issues.

• Boost energy and libido: The nutrients in the yogurt, granola, and berries can help increase energy and sexual function

69. Kimchi Fried Rice

Ingredient:

• 2 cups cooked short•grain rice, chilled
• 1 cup chopped kimchi
• 2 tbsp kimchi juice
• 1 tbsp sesame oil
• 2 eggs, beaten
• 2 green onions, chopped
• 1 tsp sesame seeds
• Salt and pepper to taste

Instructions:

1. Heat the sesame oil in a large skillet or wok over medium•high heat.

2. Add the chopped kimchi and kimchi juice. Stir•fry for 2•3 minutes until fragrant.

3. Add the chilled rice and stir•fry for 3•4 minutes, breaking up any clumps, until the rice is heated through.

4. Push the rice mixture to the side of the pan and pour the beaten eggs into the empty space. Scramble the eggs for 1•2 minutes. Combine the eggs with the rice mixture and stir to combine.

5. Remove from heat and stir in the chopped green onions and sesame seeds. Season with salt and pepper to taste.Serve hot.

For men specifically, this kimchi fried rice can help:

• Improve testosterone levels: The probiotics in the kimchi may help increase testosterone production.

• Reduce inflammation: The anti•inflammatory compounds in the sesame oil and the antioxidants in the kimchi can help reduce inflammation, which is important for men's health.

• Support prostate health: The probiotics and antioxidants in this dish may help prevent prostate issues.

• Boost energy and libido: The nutrients in the kimchi, rice, and eggs can help increase energy and sexual function.

70. Fermented Salsa

Ingredient:
- 4 medium tomatoes, diced
- 1 onion, diced
- 2 jalapeños, seeded and diced
- 3 cloves garlic, minced
- 1 tbsp sea salt
- 1 cup filtered water

Instructions:
1. In a large bowl, combine the diced tomatoes, onion, jalapeños, and minced garlic.

2. Dissolve the sea salt in the filtered water to create a brine.

3. Pour the brine over the vegetable mixture and stir to combine. The vegetables should be fully submerged in the brine.

4. Transfer the salsa mixture to a clean, wide•mouth mason jar, pressing down to remove any air pockets.

5. Cover the jar with an airlock lid or a regular lid with a small gap to allow gases to escape during fermentation.

6. Let the salsa ferment at room temperature (65•75°F) for 3•5 days, checking daily and skimming off any scum that forms.

7. Once the salsa has reached your desired level of sourness, transfer the jar to the refrigerator. The fermentation will slow down at the cooler temperature.

8. Enjoy the fermented salsa as a dip, topping, or condiment. It will keep for several months in the fridge.

Why fermented salsa supports gut health for men:
- The fermentation process increases the probiotic content of the salsa, providing beneficial bacteria for the gut.

- Tomatoes are a good source of fiber, which helps promote regular bowel movements and a healthy gut microbiome.

- Jalapeños and garlic contain antimicrobial and anti•inflammatory compounds that can help balance gut flora and reduce inflammation.

71. Chickpea and Spinach Stew

Ingredient:

• 1 tbsp olive oil
• 1 onion, diced
• 3 cloves garlic, minced
• 1 tsp ground cumin
• 1 tsp paprika
• 1/4 tsp cayenne pepper (optional)
• 1 (15oz) can chickpeas, drained and rinsed
• 1 (14oz) can diced tomatoes
• 4 cups fresh spinach, chopped
• 1 cup vegetable broth
• Salt and pepper to taste
• Chopped parsley for garnish (optional)

Instructions:

1. In a large pot or Dutch oven, heat the olive oil over medium heat. Add the diced onion and sauté for 5 minutes until translucent.

2. Add the minced garlic, cumin, paprika, and cayenne (if using). Stir and cook for 1 minute until fragrant.

3. Add the drained and rinsed chickpeas, diced tomatoes, chopped spinach, and vegetable broth. Stir to combine.

4. Bring the stew to a simmer and let it cook for 10•15 minutes, until the spinach is wilted and the flavors have melded.

5. Season with salt and pepper to taste. Serve the chickpea and spinach stew warm, garnished with chopped parsley if desired.

For men specifically, this chickpea and spinach stew can help:

• Improve testosterone levels: The fiber and nutrients in the chickpeas and spinach may help increase testosterone production.

• Reduce inflammation: The anti•inflammatory compounds in the spices and vegetables can help reduce inflammation, which is important for men's health.

This hearty and flavorful stew is a great way for men to incorporate more gut•supporting foods into their diet. Feel free to adjust the spices or add other vegetables to your liking.

72. Grilled Portobello Mushrooms

Ingredient:

• 4 large portobello mushroom caps, stems removed
• 2 tbsp olive oil
• 2 tbsp balsamic vinegar
• 2 cloves garlic, minced
• 1 tsp dried thyme
• Salt and pepper to taste

Instructions:

1. Preheat your grill or grill pan to medium•high heat.

2. In a shallow dish, whisk together the olive oil, balsamic vinegar, minced garlic, and dried thyme. Season with salt and pepper.

3. Add the portobello mushroom caps to the marinade, making sure to coat both sides evenly. Let them marinate for 10•15 minutes.

4. Grill the mushrooms for 4•5 minutes per side, until they are tender and have grill marks. Baste with any remaining marinade while grilling.

5. Transfer the grilled portobello mushrooms to a serving plate. Serve warm.

Tips:
• You can also bake the marinated mushrooms in the oven at 400°F for 15•20 minutes, flipping halfway.

• Try stuffing the grilled portobellos with cheese, roasted veggies, or breadcrumbs for a heartier meal.

• Pair the grilled portobellos with a salad, rice, or crusty bread for a complete vegetarian dish.

• Leftover grilled portobellos make great sandwich fillings or toppings for burgers.

The meaty texture and savory•sweet flavor of grilled portobello mushrooms make them a delicious and versatile vegetarian option. Enjoy!

73. Eggplant Parmesan

Ingredient:

- 2 medium eggplants, sliced into 1/2•inch thick rounds
- 1 cup all•purpose flour
- 2 eggs, beaten
- 2 cups breadcrumbs
- 1 cup grated Parmesan cheese
- 2 cups marinara sauce
- 2 cups shredded mozzarella cheese
- Fresh basil leaves for garnish

Instructions:

1. Preheat oven to 375°F. Lightly grease a 9x13 inch baking dish.

2. Set up a breading station with the flour, beaten eggs, and breadcrumbs mixed with Parmesan cheese in separate shallow dishes.

3. Dip the eggplant slices first in the flour, then the egg, and finally the breadcrumb•Parmesan mixture, coating both sides.

4. Arrange the breaded eggplant slices in a single layer in the prepared baking dish.

5. Bake for 20 minutes, then flip the eggplant slices and bake for another 15•20 minutes until golden brown.

6. Remove the eggplant from the oven and top with the marinara sauce and shredded mozzarella cheese.

7. Return to the oven and bake for an additional 15•20 minutes, until the cheese is melted and bubbly. Garnish with fresh basil leaves before serving.

For men specifically, this eggplant parmesan dish can help:

- Improve testosterone levels: The fiber and nutrients in the eggplant and the probiotics in the Parmesan cheese may help increase testosterone production.

- Reduce inflammation: The antioxidants in the marinara sauce and the anti•inflammatory properties of the eggplant can help reduce inflammation, which is important for men's health

74. Stuffed Bell Peppers with Brown Rice

Ingredient:

- 4 large bell peppers (any color)
- 1 cup cooked brown rice
- 1 lb ground turkey or lean ground beef
- 1 small onion, diced
- 3 cloves garlic, minced
- 1 (15 oz) can diced tomatoes
- 1 tsp dried oregano
- 1 tsp dried basil
- 1/2 tsp red pepper flakes (optional)
- 1 cup shredded mozzarella cheese
- Salt and pepper to taste

Instructions:

1. Preheat oven to 375°F.

2. Cut the tops off the bell peppers and remove the seeds and membranes. Place the peppers in a baking dish.

3. In a skillet over medium heat, cook the ground turkey/beef, onion, and garlic until browned and cooked through. Drain any excess fat.

4. Stir in the cooked brown rice, diced tomatoes, oregano, basil, and red pepper flakes (if using). Season with salt and pepper.

5. Stuff the mixture into the hollowed•out bell peppers. Top with the shredded mozzarella cheese.

6. Bake for 25•30 minutes, until the peppers are tender and the cheese is melted and bubbly. Serve the stuffed bell peppers warm.

Why this dish supports gut health for men:

• Brown rice is a whole grain that is high in fiber, which helps promote healthy digestion and bowel function.

• Ground turkey or beef provides protein, which is important for gut lining repair and maintenance.

• Bell peppers are rich in vitamins, minerals, and antioxidants that can help reduce inflammation in the gut. The combination of fiber, protein, and anti•inflammatory nutrients makes this a gut•friendly meal for men.

This stuffed bell pepper dish is a delicious and nutritious way for men to support their overall gut health. The fiber, protein, and other beneficial compounds work together to nourish the digestive system.

75. Tofu Scramble with Vegetables

Ingredient:

- 1 block of firm or extra•firm tofu, crumbled
- 1 tbsp olive oil
- 1 onion, diced
- 1 bell pepper, diced
- 1 cup sliced mushrooms
- 2 cups baby spinach
- 2 cloves garlic, minced
- 1 tsp turmeric
- 1 tsp cumin
- 1/2 tsp smoked paprika
- Salt and pepper to taste
- 2 tbsp nutritional yeast (optional)

Instructions:

1. Heat the olive oil in a large skillet over medium heat. Add the diced onion and sauté for 3•4 minutes until translucent.

2. Add the diced bell pepper, sliced mushrooms, and minced garlic. Sauté for another 5 minutes until the vegetables are tender.

3. Crumble the tofu into the skillet and stir to combine with the vegetables.

4. Add the turmeric, cumin, smoked paprika, salt, and pepper. Stir well to coat the tofu and vegetables.

5. Stir in the baby spinach and cook for 2•3 minutes until the spinach is wilted.

6. If using, sprinkle the nutritional yeast over the tofu scramble and stir to incorporate.

7. Serve the tofu scramble warm, garnished with extra spinach or chopped herbs if desired.

This flavorful and nutrient•dense tofu scramble is a great way for men to incorporate more gut•supporting foods into their diet. Feel free to adjust the vegetables or spices to your liking. Enjoy!

76. Veggie Burger with Avocado

Ingredient:

• 1 (15oz) can black beans, drained and rinsed
• 1 cup cooked quinoa
• 1/2 cup rolled oats
• 1/4 cup breadcrumbs
• 1 egg, beaten
• 1 tsp cumin
• 1 tsp chili powder
• 1/2 tsp garlic powder
• Salt and pepper to taste
• 4 whole wheat burger buns
• 1 avocado, sliced
• Lettuce, tomato, onion, and any other desired toppings

Instructions:

1. In a large bowl, mash the black beans with a fork or potato masher until slightly chunky.

2. Add the cooked quinoa, rolled oats, breadcrumbs, beaten egg, cumin, chili powder, garlic powder, salt, and pepper. Mix well until fully combined.

3. Divide the mixture into 4 equal patties, shaping them into burger shapes.

4. Heat a large skillet or grill pan over medium heat. Cook the veggie patties for 4•5 minutes per side, until lightly browned and heated through. Toast the burger buns.

5. Place the veggie patties on the toasted buns and top with sliced avocado, lettuce, tomato, onion, and any other desired toppings.

For men specifically, this veggie burger with avocado can help:
• Improve testosterone levels: The fiber, protein, and healthy fats in the ingredients may help increase testosterone production.

• Reduce inflammation: The anti•inflammatory properties of the avocado and other plant•based ingredients can help reduce inflammation, which is important for men's health.

• Support prostate health: The antioxidants and fiber in this dish may help prevent prostate issues.

77. Lentil and Vegetable Shepherd's Pie

Ingredient:

For the Filling:
- 1 cup brown or green lentils, rinsed
- 3 cups vegetable broth
- 1 tbsp olive oil
- 1 onion, diced
- 3 carrots, peeled and diced
- 2 celery stalks, diced
- 3 cloves garlic, minced
- 1 tsp dried thyme

Instructions:

1. Preheat oven to 375°F.

2. In a medium saucepan, combine the lentils and vegetable broth. Bring to a boil, then reduce heat and simmer for 20•25 minutes, until lentils are tender. Drain any excess liquid.

3. In a large skillet, heat the olive oil over medium heat. Add the diced onion, carrots, and celery. Sauté for 5•7 minutes until vegetables are softened.

4. Add the minced garlic, dried thyme, and dried rosemary. Cook for 1 minute until fragrant.

5. Stir in the cooked lentils and season with salt and pepper to taste.

6. Transfer the lentil and vegetable mixture to a 9x13 inch baking dish.

7. In a medium saucepan, cover the cubed potatoes with water and bring to a boil. Reduce heat and simmer for 15•20 minutes until potatoes are tender. Drain and mash with the almond milk and butter. Season with salt and pepper.

8. Spread the mashed potatoes over the lentil and vegetable filling in the baking dish. Bake for 25•30 minutes, until the potatoes are lightly browned. Let cool for 5•10 minutes before serving.

78. Zucchini Noodles with Pesto

Ingredient:

• 3 medium zucchinis, spiralized or julienned into noodles
• 1 cup fresh basil leaves
• 1/4 cup pine nuts
• 2 cloves garlic
• 1/4 cup grated Parmesan cheese
• 2 tbsp olive oil
• 1 tbsp lemon juice
• Salt and pepper to taste

Instructions:

1. In a food processor or blender, combine the basil leaves, pine nuts, garlic, Parmesan cheese, olive oil, and lemon juice. Blend until a smooth pesto forms. Season with salt and pepper to taste.

2. In a large bowl, toss the zucchini noodles with the prepared pesto until evenly coated.

3. Serve the zucchini noodles with pesto immediately, garnished with extra Parmesan cheese or pine nuts if desired.

Why is this a good gut health option for men?

1. Zucchini: Zucchini is a great source of fiber, which helps feed the beneficial bacteria in the gut. A healthy gut microbiome is important for overall health, including immune function, nutrient absorption, and even mental well•being.

2. Basil: Basil is rich in antioxidants and has anti•inflammatory properties, which can help support a healthy gut.

3. Pine nuts: Pine nuts contain healthy fats and are a good source of magnesium, which can help reduce inflammation.

4. Parmesan cheese: Parmesan cheese contains probiotics, which are live, beneficial bacteria that can help support a healthy gut.

This light and flavorful zucchini noodle dish is a great way for men to incorporate more gut•supporting foods into their diet. Feel free to adjust the ingredients to your taste preferences. Enjoy!

79. Cauliflower Tacos

Ingredient:

- 1 head of cauliflower, cut into florets
- 2 tbsp olive oil
- 1 tsp chili powder
- 1 tsp cumin
- 1/2 tsp garlic powder
- Salt and pepper to taste
- 8•10 small corn or flour tortillas
- 1 cup shredded cabbage or slaw mix
- 1 avocado, sliced
- 1/4 cup crumbled feta or queso fresco
- Chopped cilantro for garnish
- Lime wedges for serving

Instructions:

1. Preheat your oven to 400°F. Line a baking sheet with parchment paper.

2. In a large bowl, toss the cauliflower florets with the olive oil, chili powder, cumin, garlic powder, salt, and pepper until evenly coated.

3. Spread the seasoned cauliflower in a single layer on the prepared baking sheet. Roast for 20•25 minutes, stirring halfway, until the cauliflower is tender and lightly browned.

4. Warm the tortillas according to package instructions.

5. To assemble the tacos, place some of the roasted cauliflower in each tortilla. Top with shredded cabbage, sliced avocado, crumbled feta or queso fresco, and chopped cilantro.

6. Serve the cauliflower tacos immediately with lime wedges on the side.

For men specifically, these cauliflower tacos can help:

- Improve testosterone levels: The fiber, nutrients, and healthy fats in the ingredients may help increase testosterone production.

- Reduce inflammation: The anti•inflammatory compounds in the spices, cauliflower, and avocado can help reduce inflammation, which is important for men's health.

These flavorful and nutritious cauliflower tacos are a great way for men to incorporate more gut•supporting foods into their diet. Enjoy!

80. Vegetable and Quinoa Stuffed Acorn Squash

Ingredient:

• 2 acorn squash, halved and seeded
• 1 cup cooked quinoa
• 1 cup diced bell peppers
• 1 cup diced mushrooms
• 1/2 cup diced onion
• 2 cloves garlic, minced
• 1 tsp dried thyme
• 1 tsp dried rosemary
• Salt and pepper to taste
• 1/4 cup grated Parmesan cheese (optional)

Instructions:

1. Preheat oven to 400°F. Place the acorn squash halves cut•side down on a baking sheet. Bake for 30•40 minutes, until tender when pierced with a fork.

2. In a large skillet, sauté the diced bell peppers, mushrooms, and onion in a bit of olive oil over medium heat for 5•7 minutes, until softened.

3. Add the minced garlic, dried thyme, and dried rosemary. Cook for 1 minute until fragrant.

4. Stir in the cooked quinoa and season with salt and pepper to taste.

5. Flip the baked acorn squash halves over and scoop the quinoa and vegetable mixture into the cavities.

6. If using, sprinkle the grated Parmesan cheese over the top.

7. Return the stuffed squash to the oven and bake for an additional 10•15 minutes, until the cheese is melted and lightly browned. Serve the vegetable and quinoa stuffed acorn squash warm.

For men specifically, this vegetable and quinoa stuffed acorn squash can help:

• Improve testosterone levels: The fiber, protein, and nutrients in the quinoa, vegetables, and squash may help increase testosterone production.

• Reduce inflammation: The anti•inflammatory compounds in the herbs and vegetables can help reduce inflammation, which is important for men's health.

81. Baked Salmon with Dill Sauce

Ingredient:

For the Salmon:
• 4 (6 oz) salmon fillets
• 2 tbsp olive oil
• 1 tsp lemon zest
• Salt and pepper to taste

For the Dill Sauce:
• 1 cup plain Greek yogurt
• 2 tbsp chopped fresh dill
• 1 tbsp lemon juice
• 1 clove garlic, minced
• 1/4 tsp salt

Instructions:

1. Preheat your oven to 400°F. Line a baking sheet with parchment paper.

2. Place the salmon fillets on the prepared baking sheet. Drizzle with olive oil and sprinkle with lemon zest, salt, and pepper.

3. Bake the salmon for 12•15 minutes, until it flakes easily with a fork.

4. While the salmon is baking, make the dill sauce. In a small bowl, mix together the Greek yogurt, chopped dill, lemon juice, minced garlic, and salt. Serve the baked salmon warm, topped with the creamy dill sauce.

Why is this a good gut health option for men?

1. Salmon: Salmon is an excellent source of omega•3 fatty acids, which have anti•inflammatory properties that can benefit gut health.

2. Greek yogurt: The probiotic•rich Greek yogurt in the dill sauce helps support a healthy gut microbiome, which is important for overall health, including immune function, nutrient absorption, and even mental well•being.

3. Dill: Dill is a herb that contains compounds with antimicrobial and anti•inflammatory effects, which can help maintain a balanced gut.

This simple yet flavorful baked salmon dish is a great way for men to incorporate more gut•supporting foods into their diet. The creamy dill sauce complements the salmon perfectly. Enjoy!

82. Shrimp and Avocado Salad

Ingredient:

• 1 lb cooked shrimp, peeled and deveined
• 2 avocados, diced
• 1 cup cherry tomatoes, halved
• 1/2 red onion, thinly sliced
• 1/4 cup chopped cilantro
• 2 tbsp olive oil
• 2 tbsp lime juice
• 1 tsp Dijon mustard
• Salt and pepper to taste

Instructions:

1. In a large bowl, combine the cooked shrimp, diced avocados, cherry tomatoes, red onion, and chopped cilantro.

2. In a small bowl, whisk together the olive oil, lime juice, and Dijon mustard. Season with salt and pepper.

3. Pour the dressing over the shrimp and avocado mixture and gently toss to coat.

4. Serve the shrimp and avocado salad chilled or at room temperature.

Why is this a good gut health option for men?

1. Shrimp: Shrimp is a good source of protein, which is important for maintaining a healthy gut lining.

2. Avocado: Avocados are rich in fiber, which helps feed the beneficial bacteria in the gut. They also contain healthy fats that can help reduce inflammation.

3. Olive oil: The healthy monounsaturated fats in olive oil have anti•inflammatory properties, which can be beneficial for men's health.

4. Lime juice: Citrus fruits like limes are a good source of vitamin C, which can help support a healthy immune system and gut.

This refreshing and nutritious shrimp and avocado salad is a great way for men to incorporate more gut•supporting foods into their diet. Feel free to adjust the ingredients to your taste preferences. Enjoy!

83. Tuna Salad with Greek Yogurt

Ingredient:

• 2 (5 oz) cans of tuna, drained
• 1/2 cup plain Greek yogurt
• 2 tbsp diced celery
• 2 tbsp diced red onion
• 1 tbsp chopped fresh dill
• 1 tbsp Dijon mustard
• 1 tsp lemon juice
• Salt and pepper to taste

Instructions:

1. In a medium bowl, combine the drained tuna, Greek yogurt, diced celery, diced red onion, chopped dill, Dijon mustard, and lemon juice.

2. Stir everything together until well mixed.

3. Season the tuna salad with salt and pepper to taste. Serve the tuna salad on top of mixed greens, in a whole wheat pita, or with whole grain crackers.

For men specifically, this tuna salad with Greek yogurt can help:

• Improve testosterone levels: The protein and nutrients in the tuna and the probiotics in the yogurt may help increase testosterone production.

• Reduce inflammation: The anti•inflammatory properties of the dill and the vitamin C in the lemon juice can help reduce inflammation, which is important for men's health.

• Support prostate health: The antioxidants and other beneficial compounds in the dill and lemon juice may help prevent prostate issues.

• Boost energy and libido: The nutrients in the tuna, yogurt, and other ingredients can help increase energy and sexual function.

This simple yet flavorful tuna salad is a great way for men to incorporate more gut•supporting foods into their diet. The combination of protein, probiotics, and anti•inflammatory compounds makes it a nutritious and beneficial choice. Enjoy!

84. Grilled Mackerel with Lemon

Ingredient:

• 4 mackerel fillets, skin•on
• 2 tbsp olive oil
• 1 lemon, cut into wedges
• Salt and pepper to taste

Instructions:

1. Preheat your grill or grill pan to medium•high heat.

2. Pat the mackerel fillets dry with paper towels and season both sides generously with salt and pepper.

3. Brush the mackerel fillets lightly with olive oil on both sides.

4. Place the mackerel fillets skin•side down on the hot grill. Grill for 3•4 minutes per side, or until the fish flakes easily with a fork and the skin is crispy.

5. Transfer the grilled mackerel fillets to a serving plate. Serve immediately with the lemon wedges on the side.

6. Squeeze the lemon juice over the grilled mackerel just before serving.

The natural oiliness of mackerel pairs beautifully with the bright, tangy flavor of lemon. This simple grilled preparation allows the fresh flavors of the fish to shine. Enjoy!

85. Sardine Salad with Mixed Greens

Ingredient:

• 1 (4 oz) can of sardines in olive oil, drained and flaked
• 2 cups mixed greens (such as spinach, arugula, and kale)
• 1/2 cup cherry tomatoes, halved
• 1/4 cup sliced cucumber
• 2 tbsp chopped red onion
• 1 tbsp olive oil
• 1 tbsp lemon juice
• 1 tsp Dijon mustard
• Salt and pepper to taste

Instructions:

1. In a large salad bowl, combine the flaked sardines, mixed greens, cherry tomatoes, sliced cucumber, and chopped red onion.

2. In a small bowl, whisk together the olive oil, lemon juice, and Dijon mustard. Season with salt and pepper.

3. Drizzle the dressing over the sardine salad and toss gently to coat.

4. Serve the sardine salad immediately.

Why is this a good gut health option for men?

1. Sardines: Sardines are an excellent source of omega•3 fatty acids, which have anti•inflammatory properties that can benefit gut health.

2. Mixed greens: The spinach, arugula, and kale in this salad are all rich in fiber, which helps feed the beneficial bacteria in the gut. A healthy gut microbiome is important for overall health, including immune function, nutrient absorption, and even mental well•being.

3. Olive oil and lemon juice: The healthy fats in the olive oil and the vitamin C in the lemon juice can also help reduce inflammation in the gut.

This simple yet flavorful sardine salad is a great way for men to incorporate more gut•supporting foods into their diet. The combination of omega•3s, fiber, and anti•inflammatory compounds makes it a nutritious and beneficial choice. Enjoy!

86. Fish Tacos with Cabbage Slaw

Ingredient:

For the Fish:
• 1 lb white fish fillets (such as tilapia,
cod, or halibut), cut into 2•inch pieces
• 2 tbsp olive oil
• 1 tsp chili powder
• 1 tsp cumin
• 1/2 tsp garlic powder
• Salt and pepper to taste

For Serving:
• 8•10 small corn or flour tortillas
• Sliced avocado
• Lime wedges

For the Slaw:
• 2 cups shredded green cabbage
• 1 cup shredded red cabbage
• 1/2 cup shredded carrots
• 1/4 cup chopped cilantro
• 2 tbsp apple cider vinegar
• 1 tbsp olive oil
• 1 tsp honey
• Salt and pepper to taste

Instructions:

1. In a large bowl, toss the fish pieces with the olive oil, chili powder, cumin, garlic powder, salt, and pepper until evenly coated.

2. In a separate bowl, combine the shredded green and red cabbage, carrots, and chopped cilantro for the slaw.

3. In a small bowl, whisk together the apple cider vinegar, olive oil, honey, salt, and pepper. Pour the dressing over the slaw and toss to coat.

4. Heat a large skillet or grill pan over medium•high heat. Cook the seasoned fish pieces for 3•4 minutes per side, until opaque and flaky.

5. Warm the tortillas according to package instructions.

6. To assemble the tacos, place a few pieces of the cooked fish in each tortilla. Top with the cabbage slaw, sliced avocado, and a squeeze of lime juice. Serve the fish tacos immediately.

For men specifically, these fish tacos can help:

• Improve testosterone levels: The protein, healthy fats, and nutrients in the fish, avocado, and other ingredients may help increase testosterone production.

• Reduce inflammation: The anti•inflammatory properties of the fish, vegetables, and apple cider vinegar can help reduce inflammation, which is important for men's health.

87. Baked Trout with Herbs

Ingredient:

• 4 (6 oz) trout fillets
• 2 tbsp olive oil
• 2 tbsp chopped fresh parsley
• 2 tbsp chopped fresh dill
• 1 tbsp chopped fresh thyme
• 2 cloves garlic, minced
• 1 tsp lemon zest
• Salt and pepper to taste

Instructions:

1. Preheat your oven to 400°F. Line a baking sheet with parchment paper.

2. Place the trout fillets on the prepared baking sheet.

3. In a small bowl, mix together the olive oil, chopped parsley, dill, thyme, minced garlic, and lemon zest. Season with salt and pepper.

4. Spoon the herb mixture evenly over the top of the trout fillets, making sure to coat them completely.

5. Bake the trout for 12•15 minutes, until it flakes easily with a fork. Serve the baked trout warm, garnished with any extra chopped herbs if desired.

For men specifically, this baked trout with herbs can help:

• Improve testosterone levels: The omega•3s in the trout and the nutrients in the herbs may help increase testosterone production.

• Reduce inflammation: The anti•inflammatory properties of the trout, herbs, and garlic can help reduce inflammation, which is important for men's health.

• Support prostate health: The antioxidants and other beneficial compounds in the herbs may help prevent prostate issues.

The combination of omega•3•rich trout, gut•supporting herbs, and prebiotic garlic makes this a great option for men looking to improve their overall health and well•being. Enjoy this flavorful and nutritious baked trout dish!

88. Seafood Paella with Brown Rice

Ingredient:

• 1 cup short•grain brown rice
• 2 cups low•sodium chicken or vegetable broth
• 1 tbsp olive oil
• 1 onion, diced
• 3 cloves garlic, minced
• 1 tsp smoked paprika
• 1/2 tsp saffron threads (optional)
• 1 cup diced tomatoes
• 1 lb shrimp, peeled and deveined
• 1 lb mussels, scrubbed and debearded
• 1 cup frozen peas
• 2 tbsp chopped fresh parsley
• Salt and pepper to taste

Instructions:

1. In a medium saucepan, bring the brown rice and broth to a boil. Reduce heat, cover and simmer for 40•45 minutes, until rice is tender. Fluff with a fork.

2. In a large skillet or paella pan, heat the olive oil over medium heat. Add the diced onion and sauté for 5 minutes until translucent.

3. Stir in the minced garlic, smoked paprika, and saffron (if using). Cook for 1 minute until fragrant.

4. Add the diced tomatoes and their juices. Simmer for 5 minutes.

5. Nestle the shrimp and mussels into the tomato mixture. Cover and cook for 5•7 minutes, until the shrimp are opaque and the mussels have opened up.

6. Stir in the cooked brown rice and frozen peas. Cook for 2•3 minutes until heated through.

7. Remove from heat and stir in the chopped parsley. Season with salt and pepper to taste. Serve the seafood paella immediately.

This flavorful and nutritious seafood paella is a great way for men to incorporate more gut•supporting foods into their diet. Enjoy!

89. Scallops with Garlic and Lemon

Ingredient:

- 1 lb sea scallops, patted dry
- 2 tbsp olive oil
- 3 cloves garlic, minced
- 2 tbsp freshly squeezed lemon juice
- 2 tbsp unsalted butter
- 2 tbsp chopped fresh parsley
- Salt and pepper to taste

Instructions:

1. Season the scallops all over with salt and pepper.

2. Heat the olive oil in a large skillet over medium•high heat.

3. When the oil is hot, add the scallops in a single layer and sear for 2•3 minutes per side, until golden brown. Transfer the seared scallops to a plate.

4. Reduce the heat to medium and add the minced garlic to the skillet. Cook for 1 minute, stirring constantly, until fragrant.

5. Add the lemon juice and butter to the skillet. Whisk continuously until the butter is melted and the sauce is emulsified.

6. Return the seared scallops and any accumulated juices to the skillet. Toss to coat the scallops in the garlic•lemon sauce.

7. Remove from heat and stir in the chopped parsley.

8. Serve the scallops immediately, spooning the garlic•lemon sauce over the top.

The bright, garlicky lemon sauce complements the sweet, tender scallops perfectly. This dish makes a quick and elegant seafood meal.

90. Cod with Tomato and Basil

Ingredient:

• 4 cod fillets (about 1 lb total)
• 2 tbsp olive oil
• 1 pint cherry or grape tomatoes, halved
• 3 cloves garlic, minced
• 1/4 cup fresh basil leaves, chopped
• 1 tbsp balsamic vinegar
• Salt and pepper to taste

Instructions:

1. Preheat your oven to 400°F (200°C).

2. Season the cod fillets all over with salt and pepper.

3. In a large oven•safe skillet or baking dish, heat the olive oil over medium heat.

4. Add the cod fillets and sear for 2•3 minutes per side until lightly browned.

5. Remove the skillet from the heat and scatter the halved tomatoes, minced garlic, and chopped basil around the cod fillets.

6. Drizzle the balsamic vinegar over the top.

7. Transfer the skillet to the preheated oven and bake for 12•15 minutes, until the cod is cooked through and flakes easily with a fork.

8. Serve the cod immediately, spooning the tomato•basil mixture over the top.

The sweet, juicy tomatoes and fragrant basil create a delicious sauce that complements the mild, flaky cod. This one•pan dish is easy to prepare and makes a healthy, flavorful meal.

91. Roast Chicken with Root Vegetables

Ingredient:

• 1 whole chicken (3•4 lbs)
• 3 tbsp olive oil
• 1 lb mixed root vegetables (such as carrots, potatoes, parsnips, onions), peeled and cut into 1•inch pieces
• 4 cloves garlic, peeled and left whole
• 2 sprigs fresh thyme
• Salt and pepper to taste

Instructions:

1. Preheat your oven to 400°F (200°C).

2. Pat the chicken dry with paper towels and season the cavity and outside of the chicken generously with salt and pepper.

3. In a large roasting pan or baking dish, toss the cut root vegetables with 2 tablespoons of the olive oil. Spread the vegetables out in an even layer.

4. Place the chicken on top of the vegetables. Stuff the cavity with the whole garlic cloves and thyme sprigs.

5. Drizzle the remaining 1 tablespoon of olive oil over the top of the chicken.

6. Roast the chicken and vegetables in the preheated oven for 60•75 minutes, until the chicken is cooked through and the juices run clear when pierced with a knife. The internal temperature should reach 165°F (75°C).

7. Transfer the chicken to a cutting board and let it rest for 10 minutes before carving.

8. Meanwhile, give the roasted vegetables a stir in the pan juices.

9. Serve the roast chicken alongside the roasted root vegetables. Enjoy!

The chicken bastes the vegetables as it roasts, creating a delicious, caramelized medley of flavors. This one•pan meal is perfect for a cozy, comforting dinner.

92. Grilled Lamb Chops with Rosemary

Ingredient:

• 8 lamb chops (about 1•inch thick)
• 2 tbsp olive oil
• 2 tbsp chopped fresh rosemary
• 2 cloves garlic, minced
• 1 tsp salt
• 1/2 tsp black pepper

Instructions:

1. In a shallow dish, combine the olive oil, chopped rosemary, minced garlic, salt, and pepper. Add the lamb chops and turn to coat both sides evenly with the marinade.

2. Cover the dish and let the lamb chops marinate in the refrigerator for 30 minutes to 1 hour.

3. Preheat your grill or grill pan to medium•high heat.

4. Grill the lamb chops for 4•5 minutes per side, or until they reach your desired level of doneness. Use tongs to flip the chops rather than a fork to prevent losing any juices.

5. Transfer the grilled lamb chops to a serving platter and let them rest for 5 minutes before serving.

For men specifically, this grilled lamb chops with rosemary dish can help:

• Improve testosterone levels: The protein and nutrients in the lamb may help increase testosterone production.

• Reduce inflammation: The anti•inflammatory compounds in the rosemary can help reduce inflammation, which is important for men's health.

• Support prostate health: The antioxidants and other beneficial compounds in the rosemary and garlic may help prevent prostate issues.

• Boost energy and libido: The nutrients in the lamb, rosemary, and garlic can help increase energy and sexual function.

The combination of protein•rich lamb, anti•inflammatory rosemary, and gut•supporting garlic makes this a great option for men looking to support their overall health and well•being. Enjoy this flavorful and nutritious grilled lamb dish!

93. Beef and Vegetable Stir•Fry

Ingredient:

• 1 lb beef sirloin, thinly sliced
• 2 tbsp coconut oil
• 1 red bell pepper, sliced
• 1 cup broccoli florets
• 1 cup sliced mushrooms
• 1 cup snow peas
• 3 cloves garlic, minced

• 1 tbsp grated fresh ginger
• 2 tbsp coconut aminos (or low•sodium soy sauce)
• 1 tbsp apple cider vinegar
• 1 tsp sesame oil
• Salt and pepper to taste
• Chopped green onions for garnish (optional)

Instructions:

1. Heat the coconut oil in a large wok or skillet over high heat.

2. Add the beef and stir•fry for 2•3 minutes until browned. Remove the beef from the wok and set aside.

3. Add the bell pepper, broccoli, mushrooms, and snow peas to the wok. Stir•fry for 3•4 minutes until the vegetables are crisp•tender.

4. Add the garlic and ginger to the wok and cook for 1 minute, until fragrant.

5. Return the beef to the wok and add the coconut aminos, apple cider vinegar, and sesame oil. Toss everything together and cook for 2•3 minutes more.

6. Season with salt and pepper to taste. Serve the beef and vegetable stir•fry over steamed brown rice or cauliflower rice. Garnish with chopped green onions if desired.

Why is this recipe good for gut health in men?

The variety of vegetables in this stir•fry provide a range of fiber, vitamins, and minerals that support a healthy gut microbiome. The broccoli, mushrooms, and snow peas are particularly beneficial for gut health.

The coconut aminos and apple cider vinegar add probiotics and enzymes that can aid digestion and reduce inflammation in the gut.

Ginger is a natural anti•inflammatory that can help soothe the digestive system and promote better gut function.

The lean beef provides protein, which is important for maintaining a healthy gut lining and supporting overall gut health.

94. Turkey Chili with Beans

Ingredient:

• 1 lb ground turkey
• 1 tbsp olive oil
• 1 onion, diced
• 3 cloves garlic, minced
• 2 tbsp chili powder
• 1 tsp ground cumin
• 1 tsp dried oregano
• 1/2 tsp smoked paprika
• 1/4 tsp cayenne pepper (optional)
• 1 (15 oz) can diced tomatoes
• 1 (15 oz) can kidney beans, rinsed and drained
• 1 (15 oz) can black beans, rinsed and drained
• 1 cup low•sodium chicken or vegetable broth
• Salt and pepper to taste
• Chopped cilantro for garnish (optional)

Instructions:

1. In a large pot or Dutch oven, heat the olive oil over medium•high heat. Add the ground turkey and cook, breaking it up with a wooden spoon, until browned, about 5•7 minutes.

2. Add the diced onion and minced garlic to the pot. Cook for 2•3 minutes, until the onion is translucent.

3. Stir in the chili powder, cumin, oregano, smoked paprika, and cayenne (if using). Cook for 1 minute to toast the spices.

4. Pour in the diced tomatoes, kidney beans, black beans, and chicken/vegetable broth. Stir to combine.

5. Bring the chili to a simmer and let it cook for 20•25 minutes, stirring occasionally, until the flavors have melded and the chili has thickened.

6. Season with salt and pepper to taste. Serve the turkey chili hot, garnished with chopped cilantro if desired. Enjoy!

Overall, this Turkey Chili with Beans is a delicious and gut•friendly meal that can support a healthy digestive system for men.

95. Pork Tenderloin with Apple Sauce

Ingredient:

- 1 lb pork tenderloin
- 2 tbsp olive oil
- 1 tsp salt
- 1/2 tsp black pepper
- 2 apples, peeled, cored and diced
- 1/4 cup apple cider or juice
- 2 tbsp brown sugar
- 1 tsp ground cinnamon
- 1 tbsp unsalted butter

Instructions:

1. Preheat your oven to 400°F (200°C).

2. Pat the pork tenderloin dry and season all over with the salt and pepper.

3. Heat the olive oil in a large oven•safe skillet over medium•high heat. Sear the pork on all sides until browned, about 2•3 minutes per side.

4. Transfer the skillet to the preheated oven and roast the pork for 15•20 minutes, until it reaches an internal temperature of 145°F (63°C).

5. Remove the pork from the oven and let it rest for 5•10 minutes before slicing.

6. While the pork is resting, make the apple sauce. In a small saucepan, combine the diced apples, apple cider/juice, brown sugar, and cinnamon.

7. Cook over medium heat, stirring occasionally, until the apples are softened and the sauce has thickened, about 10 minutes.

8. Remove from heat and stir in the butter until melted and incorporated.

9. Slice the pork tenderloin and serve with the warm apple sauce spooned over the top.

The sweet and tangy apple sauce complements the savory pork perfectly. This dish makes for a delicious and easy weeknight meal.

96. Bison Burger with Sweet Potato

Ingredient:

- 1 lb ground bison
- 1 tsp garlic powder
- 1 tsp onion powder
- 1 tsp smoked paprika
- 1/2 tsp salt
- 1/4 tsp black pepper
- 2 medium sweet potatoes, peeled and sliced into 1/2•inch rounds
- 2 tbsp olive oil
- 4 whole wheat buns
- Lettuce, tomato, and any other desired toppings

For the Gut•Friendly Sauce:

- 1/2 cup plain Greek yogurt
- 2 tbsp apple cider vinegar
- 1 tbsp honey
- 1 tsp Dijon mustard
- 1/4 tsp salt
- 1/4 tsp black pepper

Instructions:

1. Preheat your oven to 400°F (200°C).

2. In a large bowl, gently mix together the ground bison, garlic powder, onion powder, smoked paprika, salt, and pepper until just combined. Form the mixture into 4 equal•sized patties.

3. Toss the sweet potato rounds with the olive oil and spread them out on a baking sheet. Roast in the preheated oven for 20•25 minutes, flipping halfway, until tender and lightly browned.

4. Meanwhile, make the gut•friendly sauce by whisking together all the sauce ingredients in a small bowl.

5. Heat a large skillet or grill pan over medium•high heat. Cook the bison patties for 3•4 minutes per side, or until cooked through.

6. Assemble the burgers by placing a bison patty on each whole wheat bun. Top with the roasted sweet potato rounds, lettuce, tomato, and a generous drizzle of the gut•friendly sauce

97. Chicken and Vegetable Skewers

Ingredient:

- 1 lb boneless, skinless chicken breasts, cut into 1•inch cubes
- 1 red bell pepper, cut into 1•inch pieces
- 1 zucchini, cut into 1•inch rounds
- 1 red onion, cut into 1•inch pieces
- 8 oz cremini mushrooms, halved
- 2 tbsp olive oil
- 2 tbsp lemon juice
- 1 tsp dried oregano
- 1 tsp garlic powder
- 1/2 tsp salt
- 1/4 tsp black pepper
- Wooden or metal skewers

For the Gut•Friendly Yogurt Sauce:

- 1 cup plain Greek yogurt
- 1 tbsp lemon juice
- 1 tbsp chopped fresh parsley
- 1 clove garlic, minced
- 1/4 tsp salt
- 1/4 tsp black pepper

Instructions:

1. In a large bowl, combine the chicken, bell pepper, zucchini, onion, and mushrooms. Drizzle with the olive oil and lemon juice, then sprinkle with the oregano, garlic powder, salt, and pepper. Toss to coat the ingredients evenly.

2. Thread the chicken and vegetables onto the skewers, alternating the ingredients.

3. Preheat your grill or grill pan to medium•high heat.

4. Grill the skewers for 12•15 minutes, turning occasionally, until the chicken is cooked through and the vegetables are tender.

5. While the skewers are grilling, make the gut•friendly yogurt sauce. In a small bowl, whisk together the Greek yogurt, lemon juice, parsley, garlic, salt, and pepper. Serve the grilled chicken and vegetable skewers with the yogurt sauce on the side for dipping.

Why is this recipe good for gut health in men?

The variety of vegetables, including bell peppers, zucchini, onions, and mushrooms, provide a range of fiber and prebiotic compounds that can nourish the beneficial bacteria in the gut. The chicken is a lean protein source that is easy to digest and won't cause any gut irritation.

The Greek yogurt in the dipping sauce is a probiotic•rich food that can help replenish the good bacteria in the digestive system. The lemon juice and parsley in the sauce also have anti•inflammatory properties.

98. Slow Cooker Beef Stew

Ingredient:

• 2 lbs beef stew meat, cut into 1•inch cubes
• 4 cups beef broth
• 2 medium onions, diced
• 4 carrots, peeled and sliced
• 3 celery stalks, sliced
• 3 cloves garlic, minced
• 2 bay leaves
• 1 tsp dried thyme
• 1 tsp salt
• 1/2 tsp black pepper
• 2 tbsp apple cider vinegar
• 2 tbsp coconut aminos (or low•sodium soy sauce)
• 1 lb potatoes, peeled and cubed

Instructions:

1. Place the beef stew meat, beef broth, onions, carrots, celery, garlic, bay leaves, thyme, salt, and pepper in a slow cooker. Stir to combine.

2. Cover and cook on low for 7•8 hours or on high for 4•5 hours, until the beef is very tender.

3. About 30 minutes before the stew is done, stir in the apple cider vinegar, coconut aminos, and potatoes. Continue cooking until the potatoes are tender, about 30 minutes more. Remove the bay leaves before serving.

Why is this recipe good for gut health in men?

The slow cooking process helps to break down the tough beef, making it easier to digest. The vegetables, such as carrots, celery, and onions, provide fiber to support a healthy gut microbiome.

The apple cider vinegar and coconut aminos (or soy sauce) add beneficial probiotics and enzymes that can aid digestion. They also help to reduce inflammation in the gut.

Potatoes are a good source of resistant starch, which acts as a prebiotic to feed the beneficial bacteria in the gut. This can help to improve overall gut health.

Overall, this Slow Cooker Beef Stew is a nourishing and gut•friendly meal that can support a healthy digestive system for men.

99. Grilled Steak with Chimichurri

Ingredient:

• 1 lb flank steak or skirt steak
• 2 tbsp olive oil
• Salt and pepper to taste

For the Chimichurri Sauce:
• 1 cup fresh parsley, finely chopped
• 3 cloves garlic, minced
• 1/4 cup olive oil
• 2 tbsp red wine vinegar
• 1 tbsp fresh oregano, chopped
• 1 tsp red pepper flakes
• 1/2 tsp salt
• 1/4 tsp black pepper

Instructions:

1. Make the chimichurri sauce: In a medium bowl, combine all the chimichurri ingredients and stir to mix well. Set aside.

2. Pat the steak dry and season generously with salt and pepper on both sides.

3. Preheat your grill or grill pan to high heat.

4. Drizzle the 2 tablespoons of olive oil over the steak and rub it in to coat both sides.

5. Grill the steak for 3•5 minutes per side, depending on thickness, until it reaches your desired doneness. For medium•rare, the internal temperature should be 130•135°F.

6. Transfer the grilled steak to a cutting board and let it rest for 5•10 minutes.

7. Slice the steak against the grain into thin strips.

8. Serve the grilled steak immediately, drizzled with the chimichurri sauce.

The bright, herbaceous chimichurri sauce complements the savory, charred flavor of the grilled steak perfectly. This dish makes for an easy, yet impressive, summer meal.

100. Meatloaf with Quinoa

Ingredient:

• 1 lb ground beef
• 1 cup cooked quinoa
• 1 egg, beaten
• 1/2 cup breadcrumbs
• 1/2 cup diced onion
• 2 cloves garlic, minced
• 2 tbsp ketchup
• 1 tbsp Worcestershire sauce
• 1 tsp dried oregano
• 1 tsp dried thyme
• 1/2 tsp salt
• 1/4 tsp black pepper

For the Glaze:
• 1/2 cup ketchup
• 2 tbsp brown sugar
• 1 tbsp Dijon mustard

Instructions:

1. Preheat your oven to 375°F (190°C). Grease a 9x5 inch loaf pan.

2. In a large bowl, combine the ground beef, cooked quinoa, beaten egg, breadcrumbs, onion, garlic, 2 tbsp ketchup, Worcestershire sauce, oregano, thyme, salt, and pepper. Mix until just combined, being careful not to overmix.

3. Transfer the meatloaf mixture to the prepared loaf pan and shape it into a loaf.

4. In a small bowl, whisk together the ingredients for the glaze. Spread the glaze evenly over the top of the meatloaf.

5. Bake the meatloaf for 50•60 minutes, until the internal temperature reaches 160°F (71°C). Let the meatloaf rest for 10 minutes before slicing and serving.

The addition of quinoa in this meatloaf adds extra moisture, texture, and nutritional value. Quinoa is a great source of protein, fiber, and other essential nutrients that can support overall health.

101. Chia Seed Pudding with Mango

Ingredient:

- 1/2 cup chia seeds
- 2 cups unsweetened almond milk
- 2 tbsp maple syrup
- 1 tsp vanilla extract
- 1 cup diced mango
- 2 tbsp chopped pistachios (optional)

Instructions:

1. In a medium bowl, whisk together the chia seeds, almond milk, maple syrup, and vanilla extract until well combined.

2. Cover the bowl and refrigerate for at least 4 hours, or overnight, stirring occasionally, until the chia seeds have thickened the mixture into a pudding•like consistency.

3. When ready to serve, divide the chia seed pudding into 4 bowls or jars.

4. Top each serving with 1/4 cup of diced mango.

5. Sprinkle the chopped pistachios over the top, if using.

6. Serve chilled.

Why is this recipe good for gut health in men?

Chia seeds are an excellent source of fiber, which is essential for maintaining a healthy gut. The fiber in chia seeds helps to promote regular bowel movements and can also feed the beneficial bacteria in the gut.

Mango is a great source of vitamin C, which can help to support the immune system and reduce inflammation in the gut. Mangoes also contain enzymes that can aid in digestion.

The unsweetened almond milk used in this recipe is a dairy•free option that is easy to digest and won't cause any gut irritation.

Overall, this Chia Seed Pudding with Mango is a delicious and gut•friendly breakfast or snack that can help support a healthy digestive system for men.

102. Baked Apples with Cinnamon

Ingredient:

• 4 medium•sized apples (such as Honeycrisp, Gala, or Fuji)
• 1/4 cup brown sugar
• 1 tsp ground cinnamon
• 1/4 tsp ground nutmeg
• 2 tbsp unsalted butter, softened
• 1/4 cup chopped walnuts or pecans (optional)
• Vanilla ice cream or whipped cream (optional, for serving)

Instructions:

1. Preheat your oven to 375°F (190°C). Grease a baking dish or sheet with a little butter or non•stick cooking spray.

2. Wash and core the apples, leaving a small well in the center of each one. Place the apples in the prepared baking dish.

3. In a small bowl, mix together the brown sugar, cinnamon, and nutmeg. Spoon this mixture evenly into the center of each apple.

4. Top each apple with a small pat of the softened butter.

5. If using, sprinkle the chopped nuts over the top of the apples.

6. Bake for 30•40 minutes, or until the apples are tender when pierced with a fork and the filling is bubbly.

7. Remove the baked apples from the oven and let them cool for 5•10 minutes.

8. Serve the baked apples warm, with a scoop of vanilla ice cream or a dollop of whipped cream, if desired.

The sweet, cinnamon•spiced filling complements the soft, baked apples perfectly. This simple dessert is a cozy and comforting treat, especially during the fall and winter months.

You can experiment with different types of apples or add other spices, such as ginger or allspice, to the filling. Enjoy these Baked Apples with Cinnamon as a healthy and satisfying dessert.

103. Greek Yogurt with Honey and Walnuts

Ingredient:

• 1 cup plain Greek yogurt
• 1•2 tbsp honey (to taste)
• 2 tbsp chopped walnuts
• 1 tsp ground cinnamon (optional)

Instructions:

1. Scoop the Greek yogurt into a serving bowl or individual dish.

2. Drizzle the honey over the top of the yogurt, using 1•2 tablespoons depending on your desired sweetness level.

3. Sprinkle the chopped walnuts over the honey•sweetened yogurt.

4. If desired, add a light dusting of ground cinnamon over the top.

5. Serve immediately or refrigerate until ready to enjoy.

Tips:

• Use full•fat or 2% Greek yogurt for a richer, creamier texture.
• Substitute other nuts, such as almonds or pecans, if desired.
• Add a handful of fresh berries, such as blueberries or raspberries, for extra flavor and nutrition.
• For a sweeter version, use a flavored Greek yogurt instead of plain.
• Prepare this dish in advance and store it in the refrigerator for a quick, healthy breakfast or snack.

The benefits of this Greek Yogurt with Honey and Walnuts include:

• Protein and probiotics from the Greek yogurt to support gut health
• Healthy fats and antioxidants from the walnuts
• Natural sweetness and antibacterial properties from the honey
• Potential anti•inflammatory benefits from the cinnamon (optional)

This simple, yet delicious, yogurt parfait makes for a nutritious and satisfying breakfast, snack, or dessert. The combination of creamy yogurt, sweet honey, and crunchy walnuts creates a well•balanced and flavorful dish.

104. Berry and Almond Crumble

Ingredient:

• 4 cups mixed berries (such as blueberries, raspberries, and blackberries)
• 2 tbsp granulated sugar
• 1 tbsp cornstarch
• 1 tsp vanilla extract

Crumble Topping Ingredients:
• 1 cup old•fashioned rolled oats
• 1/2 cup sliced almonds
• 1/4 cup all•purpose flour
• 1/4 cup brown sugar
• 1/4 cup unsalted butter, softened
• 1/4 tsp ground cinnamon
• 1/4 tsp salt

Instructions:

1. Preheat your oven to 375°F (190°C). Grease an 8x8 inch baking dish.

2. In a large bowl, gently toss the mixed berries with the granulated sugar, cornstarch, and vanilla extract. Transfer the berry mixture to the prepared baking dish.

3. In a separate bowl, make the crumble topping. Combine the rolled oats, sliced almonds, all•purpose flour, brown sugar, softened butter, cinnamon, and salt. Mix until the mixture resembles coarse crumbs.

4. Sprinkle the crumble topping evenly over the berry filling.

5. Bake for 30•35 minutes, or until the topping is golden brown and the berry filling is bubbling. Allow the crumble to cool for at least 15 minutes before serving. Serve warm, with a scoop of vanilla ice cream or a dollop of whipped cream, if desired.

The combination of juicy, sweet berries and the crunchy, nutty crumble topping makes this Berry and Almond Crumble a delightful and satisfying dessert. The almonds add a lovely texture and flavor to the topping.

You can use a variety of berries, such as strawberries, blueberries, raspberries, or blackberries, depending on your preference and what's in season. Enjoy this crumble as a comforting and wholesome treat.

105. Dark Chocolate Avocado Mousse

Ingredient:

- 2 ripe avocados, pitted and flesh scooped out
- 1/2 cup unsweetened cocoa powder
- 1/4 cup maple syrup
- 1 tsp vanilla extract
- 1/4 tsp sea salt
- 1/4 cup unsweetened almond milk (or milk of your choice)

Instructions:

1. In a food processor or high•powered blender, combine the avocado flesh, cocoa powder, maple syrup, vanilla extract, and sea salt. Blend until smooth and creamy, scraping down the sides as needed.

2. Add the almond milk and continue blending until the mixture is well incorporated and has a light, mousse•like texture.

3. Taste and adjust sweetness or cocoa powder to your preference.

4. Transfer the chocolate avocado mousse to individual serving dishes or a larger serving bowl.

5. Refrigerate for at least 2 hours, or until the mousse has set and chilled completely.

6. Serve the dark chocolate avocado mousse chilled, garnished with fresh berries, shaved dark chocolate, or a dusting of cocoa powder, if desired.

Tips:

- Use very ripe, soft avocados for the best texture.
- Adjust the amount of almond milk to reach your desired consistency.
- For a richer, more intense chocolate flavor, use a higher•quality cocoa powder.
- Substitute honey or agave nectar for the maple syrup, if preferred.
- Chill the mousse for at least 2 hours, but it can be made a day in advance.

This Dark Chocolate Avocado Mousse is a healthy, guilt•free dessert that's packed with nutrients. The avocado provides a creamy, velvety texture, while the cocoa powder and maple syrup create a decadent chocolate flavor.

Enjoy this nutritious and delicious mousse as a sweet treat or a healthier alternative to traditional chocolate desserts.

106. Coconut Milk Ice Cream

Ingredient:

• 2 (13.5 oz) cans full•fat coconut milk
• 3/4 cup granulated sugar
• 1/4 tsp salt
• 1 tsp vanilla extract

Instructions:

1. In a medium saucepan, whisk together the coconut milk, sugar, and salt. Heat over medium, stirring frequently, until the sugar has dissolved completely, about 5 minutes. Remove from heat and stir in the vanilla.

2. Pour the mixture into a shallow baking dish and place in the freezer. Freeze for 2 hours, stirring and scraping the edges every 30 minutes, until partially frozen.

3. Once partially frozen, transfer the mixture to a food processor or high•powered blender. Blend until smooth and creamy, about 1•2 minutes.

4. Return the blended mixture to the baking dish and freeze for another 2•3 hours, stirring and scraping the edges every 30 minutes, until fully frozen.

5. Scoop into bowls or cones and serve immediately. For a firmer texture, transfer to an airtight container and freeze for at least 4 hours or overnight before scooping.

Enjoy your homemade coconut milk ice cream! The coconut flavor really shines through.

107. Almond Flour Brownies

Ingredient:

• 1 cup (2 sticks) unsalted butter, melted
• 1 cup granulated sugar
• 3 large eggs
• 1 tsp vanilla extract
• 1/2 cup unsweetened cocoa powder
• 1 cup almond flour
• 1/4 tsp salt
• 1/2 cup dark chocolate chips (optional)

Instructions:

1. Preheat your oven to 350°F (175°C). Grease an 8x8 inch baking pan.

2. In a large bowl, whisk together the melted butter and granulated sugar until combined.

3. Add the eggs one at a time, whisking well after each addition. Stir in the vanilla extract.

4. Sift in the cocoa powder and almond flour. Add the salt and stir until just combined, being careful not to overmix.

5. Fold in the dark chocolate chips, if using.

6. Pour the brownie batter into the prepared baking pan and spread it out evenly.

7. Bake for 25•30 minutes, or until a toothpick inserted in the center comes out with a few moist crumbs attached.

8. Allow the brownies to cool completely in the pan before cutting into squares.

The almond flour in these brownies gives them a rich, fudgy texture without the need for traditional wheat flour. They are a delicious gluten•free and grain•free treat.

You can customize these brownies by adding chopped nuts, shredded coconut, or other mix•ins to the batter. Enjoy these almond flour brownies as a guilt•free indulgence.

108. Banana and Oat Cookies

Ingredient:

• 2 ripe bananas, mashed
• 1 1/2 cups rolled oats
• 1/4 cup unsweetened shredded coconut
• 1/4 cup chopped walnuts or pecans (optional)
• 1 tsp ground cinnamon
• 1/4 tsp salt

Instructions:

1. Preheat your oven to 350°F (175°C). Line a baking sheet with parchment paper.

2. In a medium bowl, mash the ripe bananas until smooth.

3. Add the rolled oats, shredded coconut, chopped nuts (if using), cinnamon, and salt. Stir until well combined.

4. Scoop the cookie dough by the tablespoonful onto the prepared baking sheet, spacing them about 2 inches apart.

5. Bake for 12•15 minutes, or until the cookies are lightly golden and set.

6. Remove the cookies from the oven and let them cool on the baking sheet for 5 minutes before transferring them to a wire rack to cool completely.

Tips:

• Use very ripe, spotty bananas for the best flavor and sweetness.
• Adjust the amount of nuts or coconut to your taste preference.
• For a chewier cookie, bake for the shorter end of the time range.
• For a crunchier cookie, bake for the longer end of the time range.
• Store the cooled cookies in an airtight container at room temperature for up to 5 days.

These Banana and Oat Cookies are a healthy, naturally sweetened treat that's perfect for a snack or breakfast. The oats provide fiber and complex carbohydrates, while the bananas and nuts offer additional nutrients and healthy fats.

These cookies are also gluten•free, dairy•free, and can be made vegan by omitting the optional nuts. Enjoy them as a guilt•free indulgence!

109. Apple and Blueberry Crisp

Ingredient:
- 4 cups peeled, cored, and sliced apples
- 2 cups fresh or frozen blueberries
- 2 tbsp granulated sugar
- 1 tbsp all•purpose flour
- 1 tsp ground cinnamon

Topping Ingredients:
- 1 cup old•fashioned rolled oats
- 1/2 cup all•purpose flour
- 1/2 cup packed brown sugar
- 1/4 cup unsalted butter, softened
- 1/4 tsp ground cinnamon
- 1/4 tsp salt

Instructions:

1. Preheat your oven to 375°F (190°C). Grease an 8x8 inch baking dish.

2. In a large bowl, combine the sliced apples, blueberries, granulated sugar, 1 tbsp flour, and 1 tsp cinnamon. Toss to coat the fruit. Transfer the fruit mixture to the prepared baking dish.

3. In a separate bowl, make the topping. Combine the rolled oats, 1/2 cup flour, brown sugar, softened butter, 1/4 tsp cinnamon, and salt. Mix until the mixture resembles coarse crumbs.

4. Sprinkle the oat topping evenly over the fruit in the baking dish.

5. Bake for 30•35 minutes, or until the fruit is bubbling and the topping is golden brown.

6. Allow the crisp to cool for at least 15 minutes before serving.

7. Serve warm, with a scoop of vanilla ice cream or a dollop of whipped cream, if desired.

The combination of sweet apples and tart blueberries creates a delicious filling, while the crunchy oat topping adds a lovely texture. This Apple and Blueberry Crisp is a comforting and satisfying dessert that's perfect for any occasion.

Congratulations on completing ***"Gut Health Cookbook for Men: 115+ Recipes to Support Digestive Harmony and Energy"!*** You've embarked on a journey to prioritize your digestive health with over 115 nourishing and flavorful recipes tailored specifically for men.

What You've Achieved

Throughout this cookbook, you've explored recipes designed not only to satisfy your taste buds but also to support your digestive system. By incorporating ingredients known for their gut-friendly properties—such as fiber, probiotics, and nutrient-rich foods—you've taken proactive steps toward enhancing your overall well-being and energy levels.

Beyond the Kitchen

Improving your digestive health extends beyond the meals you prepare. It's about adopting sustainable lifestyle practices that complement your dietary choices. Whether it's staying hydrated, managing stress, or maintaining regular physical activity, these habits work synergistically with your diet to promote digestive harmony and overall health.

Keep Exploring and Adapting

Your journey toward optimal digestive health doesn't end here. Continue to experiment with the recipes in this book, personalize them to suit your preferences, and explore new ingredients and flavors. Every meal is an opportunity to nourish your body and discover what works best for you.

Share Your Knowledge

As you continue to prioritize gut health, share your knowledge and experiences with others. Whether it's cooking for family and friends, discussing dietary choices, or advocating for digestive wellness, your journey can inspire and empower those around you to make positive changes in their own lives.

Final Thoughts

Thank you for choosing "Gut Health Cookbook for Men: 115+ Recipes to Support Digestive Harmony and Energy" as your guide to improving digestive health through delicious and nutritious meals. May the recipes and insights gathered here continue to fuel your journey toward greater well-being and vitality. Here's to a healthier digestive system and a more energized you!